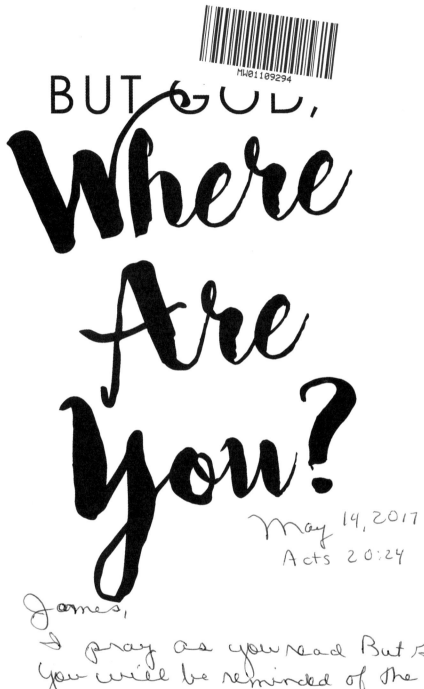

BUT GOD, Where Are You?

May 14, 2017
Acts 20:24

James,
I pray as you read But God...
you will be reminded of the
power of prayer, Gods faithfullness
and His unconditional love!

she *Believed* she could, so she did!

Blessings,
Linda
Harris

BUT GOD, Where Are You?

FINDING HOPE IN THE DIFFICULT JOURNEY THROUGH ENVIRONMENTAL ILLNESS

LINDA RANEY HARRISS, RN, LPC

WHAT PEOPLE ARE SAYING ABOUT
BUT GOD, WHERE ARE YOU?

Linda's memoir will inspire you, give you hope and ignite your faith as you read about the mighty hand of God working in her life and in the lives of those who loved and cared for her. *But God, Where Are You?* will change your life as you read Linda's incredible accounts of unconditional love and commitment in marriage and family, answered prayers, miracles, visions, and dreams.

Be ready to be encouraged and blessed while you experience the love and faithfulness of God Almighty as never before. The Lord gave me the privilege of walking with Linda and her family when she was in the middle of her severe tests of faith. I encouraged her to hang onto the truth she knew about God. By God' grace she was led to her life's work—helping other people recover from the surprises that life has brought them. So blessed!

— Frankie Rainey, Th.D.,
   Professor of Christian Studies
   Howard Payne University

With courageous transparency Linda Harriss takes her readers through the frightening harshness of some of life's darkest corners into the bright light of God's faithfulness and love. Be prepared: readers of *But God, Where Are You?* will experience their own soul-searching pinnacles of personal conviction, personal challenge, and personal victory. It is well worth the journey.

— Dr. Richard Jackson
   Pastor Emeritus, North Phoenix Baptist Church
   President, Jackson Center for Evangelism & Encouragement

ISBN: 978-0-9973372-7-3
Published by Baxter Press
First printed in 2017
Printed in the United States

Some of the names, identities, and locations mentioned in this book have been changed in order to protect privacy.

THIS BOOK IS DEDICATED TO:

My Lord and Savior, Jesus Christ—Thank you for being faithful as I traveled through "the dark night of the soul." You have turned my ashes into beauty, my grief and pain into strength, and my story for your glory. Forever grateful!

Earl—When the Lord brought us together, He had a master plan for our lives. He knew I needed a husband who would be the epitome of love, faithfulness, and commitment. You, Babe, are exemplary of a godly husband. Thank you for always believing in me and for being the wind beneath my wings. You refused to let me give up. Eternally grateful! I love you!

Mom, Rose Mary Raney—Even though you are in heaven now, I could not have made it through this journey of faith without you. Thank you for instilling a passion for Jesus in me from the time you carried me in your womb. My heart's desire is to carry on your legacy of faith and to love others as you did, through the heart and eyes of Jesus. You continue to be my inspiration!

Dad, Hughie Raney, Sr.—I'm so grateful you taught me a work ethic that never stops until the project is completed. I relied on it heavily in pursuing this dream. I love and appreciate you so much!

Christie and Greg—I'm so thankful the Lord chose me to be your mom. Out of this extremely difficult time in our lives, I have seen you both transform into godly individuals with caring hearts who know how to love and reach out to others who are hurting. You both have blessed my life more than words could ever describe. I'm so proud of you. Thank you for loving me and caring for me when I couldn't love and care for myself. Endless love!

Grandmother (Vesta Harriss), my wonderful mother-in-law—You certainly surpassed my highest hopes and expectations for a mother-in-law. You always loved me like a daughter, and your servant's heart was such a reflection of Christ. Thank you for always being there for me and our family. We couldn't have made this journey without you.

Melissa Raney, my niece—Through your nineteen years of battling a major illness, you taught me what it means to persevere and fight till the end. To this day, your joyful spirit in the midst of adversity encourages and challenges me to see every day as a gift. We all love and miss you, but will see you again someday!

TABLE OF CONTENTS

INTRODUCTION

*I consider my life worth nothing to me, if only I may finish
the race and complete the task the Lord Jesus has given me—
the task of testifying to the gospel of God's grace.*
—*Acts 20:24*

ON MAY 16, 1985, I received a medical diagnosis that would forever change my life. I had Environmental Illness, a 21th-century syndrome caused by contact with the toxic chemicals that saturate every aspect of our modern world.

My vibrant, independent life vanished. Blindsided, I suddenly found myself an invalid, bedridden, living in isolation, and fighting for my life.

The wonderful life I once lived was now nothing but a fading memory. How could this have happened to me? And where was God in the middle of my ravaged life?

Admitted to an isolation unit in a hospital in Houston, Texas, I learned that I was a Universal Reactor, severely allergic to basically my entire world—everything I could see, taste, or smell. Feeling alone and devastated, I began my descent into what seemed to be a nightmare of depression and hopelessness.

While living in isolation for fifteen months, God continually brought to my mind Hosea 4:6: "My people are destroyed by a lack of knowledge." I began to believe that He might want to use my seemingly unbelievable experience as the basis of a message that others needed to hear.

So began an incredible journey of faith during which God chose to reveal Himself in the midst of human desperation. I heard His still, small voice. I saw His power in supernatural dreams, visions, and even miracles. He tenderly ministered to me through earthly hands. Embraced by a strong Christian family, married to committed husband, loved unconditionally by two devoted children, cared for by a godly mother who constantly prayed at my bedside, a devoted mother-in-law (known as Grandmother), I was graciously restored by God.

As twenty-seven years of life intervened, the tragedy of Environmental Illness became less a daily thought and more a buried pain. Then, as I had the privilege of caring for my mother during her lengthy battle with lymphoma, I clearly understood that life runs its course in a cycle. When Mom had cared for me twenty-seven years earlier, she was unknowingly preparing me for the day that I would care for her. I came to understand and accept that whether God chooses to spare our lives or to walk with us through the valley of the shadow of death, He is a faithful and trustworthy friend.

With a triumphant voice of faith, I now could answer my own question: *But God, where are You?*

CHAPTER ONE

WHEN LIFE FALLS APART

*If only my anguish could be weighed and all my misery be
placed on the scales!*
—Job 6:2

MY LIFE IS SO PERFECT, IT'S ALMOST SCARY, I realized one crisp January dawn in 1985. From the quiet of my laundry room I slipped shirts onto hangers and counted my blessings: My husband was terrific, our two children were absolute joys, financially we were doing okay, my nursing career was satisfying, we belonged to a church full of loving Christian friends, and the home we loved sat on a hill overlooking central Texas. Who could ask for anything more?

I smiled at the breathtaking sunrise peeking over the hill. *Lord, only You and I are awake at this time of the morning.* I'd always loved being an early riser. It made me feel as if I was helping God turn on the bright lights that ushered in each new day. Closing the dryer door, I headed toward the kitchen to unload the dishwasher before leaving for work. Along the way, I peeked into our new game room.

Earl and I had decided to add this spacious area onto our house so our children—Christie, age fourteen, and Greg, age twelve—could invite their friends over and have a good time. This way, we would know who our children were with and what they were doing. Besides, we wanted a place where we could entertain young people from our church. I had been on the search committee that had just selected a new youth director, and we had offered to open our home anytime he needed a place to fellowship.

We'd put the final touches on the game room just two weeks before, and it looked great. The large "fun zone" was equipped with everything we thought our children and their friends would enjoy—a jukebox, pool table, ping pong table, and (of course) a big-screen TV. Built-in shelves held rows of old classic movies, exercise programs, and home videos of our children. The walls were covered with 16" x 24" portraits of the kids participating in their various athletic activities: track, basketball, volleyball, football, cheerleading. We had even chosen ceramic tile for the floor so visitors wouldn't have to worry about accidentally spilling refreshments.

One wall of the room was lined with lots of big windows, overlooking the volleyball poles and net we had set up on the back lawn. Beyond that, a refreshing view of the hills, trees, and wide-open spaces behind our home provided a picture-perfect backdrop. I tore my gaze from the game room and proceeded to the dressing room. Earl already had taken Christie and Greg to school, and I was putting the final touches on my hair before leaving for work.

As I peered into the mirror and brushed my hair, not really thinking about anything in particular, out of nowhere I heard a strange voice I'd never heard before. It was not audible, yet it spoke clearly and harshly as if it had been.

You're going to have to die, you're going to have to die, the voice seethed.

My heart raced. I knew Earl and the children had already left the house, but I found myself walking through each room to make sure no one had entered without my knowledge. I continued to glance around me, but saw no one. After a few moments, I calmed myself down, tried to shrug it off, and left for work. But I couldn't shake the uneasiness. It clung to me for weeks.

I'd never thought about having to die. I had no reason to die. I was healthy and had everything I wanted. What did this mean? And I couldn't tell anyone about the bizarre thing that had happened. Who would believe that I really "heard" the voice?

Finally in February, I called my friends Judy Lee and Susan Preston. "Please pray for me," I said. "I feel like God is in the process of making some changes in my life." When they asked what was going on, I simply said, "Oh, I can't explain it . . . just a feeling or something." Without further questioning, they both agreed to pray.

Symptoms Trump Self-Sufficiency

On week days I worked as a school nurse, which was both rewarding and challenging. I spent some weekends, holidays, and a few days during the summer at Brownwood Medical Center, where I had trained during nursing school. But now, a few weeks after hearing the strange voice, I began to notice strange symptoms in my body, such as shortness of breath, dizziness, sadness, mental confusion, headaches, and fatigue. I felt severe pain in my muscles and joints. Often I became sick to my stomach and started losing weight rapidly.

I didn't tell anyone I wasn't feeling well, because I didn't want to worry them. After all, I was a nurse. I should be able to take care of this problem on my own, the way I had handled every other situation in my life. Independence and pride had taken root many years ago, deep in my childhood. I was brought up with an unspoken, yet very clear, message: Be self-sufficient. Never ask for help. Believe me, I had no intention of marring the image my family had so carefully built into me.

As the weeks went by, however, my symptoms grew more severe. My weight dropped even further. I tried to deny what was happening in my body and hoped and prayed everything would just go away. Instead, I became more ill with each passing day. Pushing myself and hiding how badly I felt was becoming more and more difficult.

Early March I had been invited to speak at a Christian women's conference in Houston. During this conference, scheduled for April, I would be speaking on nutrition in relationship to health. I had always been passionate about eating healthy and welcomed opportunities to teach others about the importance of a good diet. It was exciting to be invited, but now I was uncertain about my own health.

The date finally arrived. My symptoms had gotten much worse and I wasn't sure I could make it through my presentation. I felt I could barely stand, as if my whole body was trying to shut down. But I knew the conference attendees were counting on me and I couldn't disappoint them.

Earl and the children accompanied me on the six-hour trip to Houston so we could all visit my parents, who lived nearby. We arrived at the hotel quite late and went to bed right away.

The following morning I felt so ill I didn't think I could make it out of bed. I begged the Lord to carry me through the day.

During my entire presentation, a battle raged inside me. My body ached all over. I was so tired and weak, and felt like I would pass out. I fought to hold back the tears, but managed to make it through. After the conference my family and I headed to my parents' house, where Mom had prepared a large meal for us. But when she called everyone to the table to eat, I suddenly dreaded the thought. For some time, even the smell of food made me terribly nauseated and caused my chest to tighten. But Mom had prepared my favorites—baked squash, tossed garden salad, and baked chicken. Out of appreciation and respect, I loaded up my plate. But I couldn't bring myself to eat a single bite.

As a diversionary tactic, I engaged in lively conversations with everyone. But Mom noticed my plate remained untouched. "Why aren't you eating?" she asked. "I prepared all your favorite foods."

I forced down a few bites of salad. Within seconds, I started to hyperventilate; my chest felt as though it had a tight band around it, and I was sure I was going to pass out.

"Are you sick, Linda?" Mom asked, concern etched on her face.

"Everything's fine," I assured her. I got up from the table and hurried off to another room so she couldn't quiz me anymore. I was afraid to let anyone—even my family—know that I was feeling so ill. I didn't need anyone to take care of me. That just wasn't my norm.

On Sunday morning we drove back to our home in Brownwood. The trip and the conference had really exhausted me. However, my sleep became very disturbed. I could only sleep for short periods of time. *How will I make it to work on Monday morning?* I anguished.

A Secret Revealed

Before long I was sleeping ten hours every night—twice as many as I normally needed. Day by day, my symptoms grew more intense. I experienced severe depression, increased shortness of breath, headaches, and my body twitched and ached. My excessive sleeping patterns later turned to insomnia. Several times, I had to consciously force myself to breathe. I almost passed out every time I ate anything.

Everyone noticed my extreme weight loss. When they asked about it, I simply told them I was dieting. But I knew I needed to do something soon. I felt as if my entire body was shutting down.

One day I woke up too sick to go to work and called my sister, Delores. "Pray for me," I begged. "I'm not feeling well." I didn't tell her how serious my condition was. "Promise not to tell anyone," I added. She made me agree to get medical help immediately. But I just couldn't. I was determined to take care of this problem on my own. I refused to worry anyone. Besides, if I admitted the seriousness of my problem to anyone, then I'd have to admit it to myself. I just kept telling myself that I'd come up with a solution to the problem. I just needed a little time. I couldn't admit how afraid I was and that I was losing my health. I couldn't mar my image of being strong no matter the circumstance or situation.

Maybe I'd just wake up one morning and this was just a bad dream.

A few days later my husband, Earl, told me about a new clothing store that had just opened in town. "Let's all go," he suggested, so we hopped into the car and made the short trip into town. We had only been in the building a few minutes when suddenly I could barely breathe.

"Are you all right?" Earl asked, staring at me.

"I'm okay," I panted, gasping for air. "But can we go home?"

I walked toward the exit and my legs collapsed beneath me. Earl caught me before I passed out and helped me walk. He motioned for Christie and Greg to follow us to the car.

When we got home, Earl walked me to our room and helped me into bed.

"I'm okay," I tried to assure him. "Just go back to the garage and get my purse from the car." Seeing the fear in Greg and Christie's eyes, I hurried them off to their bedrooms to do their homework. "I'll be better by morning," I promised.

I slept briefly, then woke to the muffled sounds of sobbing. Struggling to pull myself up, I stumbled down the hall to my daughter's room. She was lying on her bed, crying. I sat beside her.

"Mom, I'm scared something bad is wrong with you," she moaned. "I don't want anything to happen to you."

We prayed together, asking for God's guidance. Earl came into the room and joined us.

As I sat there on my daughter's bed, my body started to tremble. I again felt like I was going to pass out and finally confessed to my family that I had not been honest with them about my health. "I haven't been well for a couple of months or more," I admitted. For the first time, I started to cry. "I'm going to be okay, though," I assured them.

"Why didn't you tell us before?" Earl asked.

"I hated for you to worry about me."

Earl covered my hands with his. "We're going to do everything we can to get you well." He looked deep into my eyes. I knew he could see the pain and confusion there. "I'm going to take you to the hospital right now," he announced.

"I can't do that," I moaned. I didn't want the nurses and doctors at the hospital I occasionally worked with to see me sick. That ongoing family message played in my mind: Never ask for help, be self-sufficient.

"At least wait until morning," I begged. "I'll place a few phone calls to some out-of-town physicians I know, and we'll make a decision after that."

Earl didn't like the idea, but finally agreed to my wishes. I laid awake all night, hoping and praying I'd see morning. Earl kept begging me to go to the hospital, but refused to budge.

Houston Bound

By morning I was gasping for air and trembling. I felt so weak and couldn't even make a phone call. Earl contacted one of the doctors I knew in Austin, three hours away. We got an appointment to see Dr. Richards that very day. Mom came from Pearland to be with us.

My husband helped me into the car. I felt weak and lifeless and laid down in the back seat all the way to Austin. I reminded Earl that I did not want anyone to know we were going to the doctor. The family message played over and over in my mind, that any form of weakness was unacceptable. I'd rather subject myself to a road trip than risk letting someone know I was sick and didn't have it together. Earl drove quickly to make the appointment on time. All I could do was pray for safety as the car sped down the road, careening on every curve.

I briefed Dr. Richards on my symptoms. He ran an EKG and blood-sugar test, both of which resulted in normal readings. Further blood work showed I was anemic. My white blood count was low and most of my minerals were depleted. That didn't surprise me—I had been starving for quite some time because eating made me so sick.

After all the tests were completed, Dr. Richards said he believed my problem was allergy related.

"That's crazy," I responded. "I have never been allergic to anything."

He did not relent, and I was finally desperate enough to get the help I needed. So I agreed to stay and take the allergy tests.

The nurse first checked to make sure I wasn't allergic to the preservatives in the allergens used in the tests. Unfortunately I was, and started having the symptoms that had plagued me the last few months.

Dr. Richards informed me that he could not treat me. "You have more than simple allergies," he explained. "Your reaction to the allergens indicates that you are most likely chemically sensitive. In my opinion, your immune system has significant problems," he added. "I'm not sure anyone can do anything for your condition."

Earl stood and placed his hands on the doctor's desk. He spoke in a more assertive voice than I had ever heard him use. "If you can't help her," he said, "please find someone who can."

Dr. Richards told his nurse to put everything on hold. "Let me see if I can find someone." He went into his personal office and closed the door. As we sat in the examination room, panic and fear swept over me. I was terrified that I would be stuck in poor health and depression for the rest of my life. I fell into Earl's arms, weeping like a small child.

"Don't worry," he assured me, stroking my hair. "We'll find the help you need." His voice caught in his throat. "And I will always take care of you."

After several minutes, Dr. Richards returned. "Here is the phone number for a group of doctors who specialize in the immune system and the treatment of allergies." He handed me a card with the clinic's information. "The clinic uses allergens without preservatives," he explained. "So if you have an allergic reaction during testing there, the doctor will know you are reacting to the allergen itself, not just the preservatives."

We made an appointment for May 6, at 9:00 a.m. with the allergy clinic in Houston. They told us it would take up to eight days to complete the battery of tests. We were also informed that makeup, hair spray, perfume, and any clothing made of synthetic material would not be allowed in the clinic. This policy was in place to protect the chemically sensitive patients who were there.

Seeking Answers

The drive to the allergy clinic in Houston was long. Neither Mom nor I spoke much. Earl stayed home to be with the children and get caught up at work. Mom and I sat anxiously in the waiting room. Finally, I was led back to an examination room. Mom accompanied me as a nurse recorded my blood pressure, weight, and temperature. Then a tall, young man with blondish-brown hair came in and introduced himself as Dr. Morlen. He did a general assessment on me, asking the usual questions about my health history and scribbling my answers on a stack of papers attached to a clipboard.

When he was satisfied with the paperwork, Dr. Morlen directed me to the testing room. There I was injected with minute dosages of various things I might possibly be allergic to. After each test, I experienced a dramatic reaction. A severe tightness seized my head. It seemed as if the right side of my brain would literally burst through my skull. I became confused and dizzy. By the end of the first day, I was more depressed than ever.

After eight long days, there wasn't anything I was tested for that I didn't have an allergic reaction to. I left the clinic hopeless and exhausted. We drove back to my parents' house where we were staying and prepared ourselves for a long night.

A Diagnosis

I didn't sleep a wink. When the sun finally came up I was anxious to meet with Dr. Morlen and discuss the results of my tests. Mom and I dressed quickly, arriving thirty minutes early for the appointment.

When the nurse called my name, Mom and I were escorted to the examination room. Dr. Morlen came in with a distraught look on his face, causing my knees to quiver and my heart to pound out of my chest. His first question was, "Have you done anything different in your home recently?"

I immediately thought of our new game room and told him all about it.

Dr. Morlen nodded. "The chemicals in the materials you used to build that room are most likely the thing that finally overloaded your immune system, causing it to no longer function properly."

I couldn't believe what I was hearing. Surely the game room, which we had built to provide a safe place for our children and other young people, couldn't be the cause of my physical problems. "How can this happen?" I asked in a daze.

"Due to the high level of chemicals found these days in our foods, clothing, homes, workplaces, and everything else in the environment," he explained, "sometimes the human body experiences a chemical overload. The organs and various systems are no longer able to function in a healthy manner.

"Oh," was all I could manage as his words sunk in.

"You work as a school nurse. Most schools are very toxic due to the large number of chemicals used in cleaning and sanitizing, as well as, poor ventilation. Chemicals stay trapped in schools because there are no windows that open allowing fresh air in and toxins out."

But how could such a thing happen to me? I had been a nurse for three years. I knew how to take proper care of my body. I avoided junk foods, soft drinks, candy, cookies, and everything containing sugar or white flour. No one had told me that everyday building materials could affect my body in such an adverse way.

Dr. Morlen asked if I could have had any other toxic exposures in the past. I thought back to when Earl and I first built our house in 1979. Since we lived in the country, we had a few small natural-gas wells on the property. We had decided to use the natural gas from the wells to provide energy for our heating and air-conditioning units.

"I do remember an incident that happened a few months ago," I said. "When Earl was out of town on business, the gas water heater had shut off and we didn't have hot water for baths that morning. I attempted to restart the pilot light, but without success."

I explained that I took the children to school, then came back home and spent a considerable amount of time in the house. I called a neighbor, Dee England, who worked for our local gas company, and he came over to try to light the pilot. When Dee opened the door to the water heater, he noticed that the valve was open all the way and gas was spewing into the air. Since it was unscented, I hadn't realized it was on, and I'd been breathing it all that time. Dee advised me to open all the windows and leave my house until the gas could dissipate. He came back later in the day with a gas-detection meter. After several hours, he finally gave me approval to return to my home.

In March of that year after the natural-gas incident, Earl and I took a vacation to China. One night as we sat eating in a restaurant, I started shaking. I could barely breathe and felt as if I was going to faint. Earl helped me back to our hotel room, since I was not able to walk unassisted. I had to remind myself to keep breathing. My body felt strange that night, as if it was trying to shut down, yet at the same time fighting hard to live.

After I related these situations to Dr. Morlen, he explained that each exposure was part of the toxic overload. "The chemicals in the building materials for your game room began breaking down your immunities. The gas leak in your home further overloaded your system, exacerbating the problem. Your trip to China appears to have been the final straw."

"Do you think it was what we ate at the restaurant?" I asked, remembering vividly my body's response to the dinner.

"The food most likely contained preservatives," Dr. Morlen conceded, "which certainly would have brought on the dramatic symptoms. But it takes a major exposure to cause a chemical overload. It's more likely that some type of heavy pesticide was used in your hotel room, and breathing the toxic fumes set things off. At any rate, your body simply couldn't take any more."

It was all too bizarre to comprehend.

"The area of your immune system that controls allergies is now functioning at an extremely low level," continued Dr. Morlen. "While many people suffer from simple allergic reactions to a few everyday things such as pollen or dairy products, because of your chemical exposures and poorly functioning immune system, your body reacts violently . . . to everything. You have cerebral allergies. Your brain is tremendously affected by chemical exposures, which sets off various kinds of symptoms and reactions." Hearing this made me think about people who use illegal drugs and how their brains are affected by the chemicals they put into their bodies. I wondered what unresolved issues or hurts they had in their lives that made them vulnerable to using drugs. I assumed they were looking for temporary pain relief. Sadly, the downside of their coping method was that it made them susceptible to various health issues and mood disorders and perhaps even death.

Allergic to Everything

Dr. Morlen then gave us the official diagnosis. "Mrs. Harriss," he stated, "you are what we classify as a Universal Reactor. You have what we call Environmental Illness. You have cerebral reactions. People most commonly associate allergic reactions with runny noses, congestion, rashes, etc. But your reactions cause your brain to swell. Unfortunately, when that happens your body organs can be affected. It is common to have a lot of neurological symptoms such as shaking, tics, mental fogginess, mood swings, heart palpitations, and various other symptoms."

As I sat in that testing room, waiting and praying for the pain to subside, I felt completely alone.

I tried to comprehend his words, but it was hard to believe my ears.

You are extremely allergic to every kind of food, tree, mold, weed, and grass, the materials in your home, your clothing and makeup—basically everything you wear, see, touch, smell, taste, or breathe," he continued. I soon realized that people become ill with Environmental Illness and Multiple Chemical Sensitivities because the world we live in has become so toxic. All the chemicals found in our food, drink, air, cleaning supplies, pesticides, body products, businesses, industries, and many others wreak havoc on our immune systems. Our bodies cannot deal with all the toxins.

"The fragrance industry uses over 4,000 different chemicals in their products. Our bodies were not designed to handle chemicals, and after a while our immune system becomes overloaded and breaks down. When this happens you become susceptible to illness, disease, allergies, and chemical sensitivities," explained the doctor. "Unfortunately, untold people are walking around feeling miserable with numerous health problems and diseases in their bodies. And they are clueless as to what the underlying cause of their physical condition really is. Any part of your body can be affected: emotional, respiratory, gastrointestinal, skin, musculoskeletal, cardiovascular, eyes, ears, genitourinary, etc."

As surprising as this avalanche of news was, there was more to come.

"Many people have Sick Building Syndrome," said the doctor. "This illness is caused by indoor pollution which can be caused by chemicals and poor ventilation. Individuals may experience an array of symptoms when exposed to this type environment."

"So I'm allergic to everything? How can a person be allergic to everything?" I asked the doctor.

"Even those braces on your teeth," he pointed out, "will have to come off."

"My braces?" I had waited thirty-five years to have my teeth straightened!

"You are most likely allergic to the type of metal they're made of, as well as to the glue that holds them to your teeth."

Dr. Morlen excused himself and soon returned with Peggy, the nutritionist for the allergy clinic. She shook her head as she studied my test results.

"I'm going to try to work out a diet plan for you," Peggy promised, "but it won't be easy." She ranked my allergies to foods according to severity and advised me to eat only those I reacted to least. My list of "safer" foods was short. I found myself feeling so overwhelmed wondering if I would just starve to death.

A Universal Reactor

Dr. Morlen insisted I check into a hospital, which had a special "environmentally safe" ward for Universal Reactors. I didn't like this label that was being attached to me. It was too strange; it made me feel like I was from another world. I sat there speechless, trying to understand what was happening.

"How long . . ." I choked on the words. "How long would I have to stay there?"

"You'll be there at least two or three months," he answered.

Two or three months sounded like an eternity. My family needed me, even though I was not able to take care of them. And, I needed them. I didn't think I could handle being gone for so long. It would be a very difficult two or three months, and therefore I would have to think about going. I couldn't make a commitment without talking to Earl and praying.

"The hospital will provide an opportunity for your system to detox," Dr. Morlen urged. "After that, you will be taught how to create your own safe place."

"What do you mean, safe place?" The words nearly stuck in my throat.

"We will provide an evaluation and suggestions for the best way to protect yourself from the things you are allergic to. Some people live in isolation rooms in their own homes; others move to communities that are less toxic and safer for Universal Reactors."

My heart skipped a beat. "But . . . eventually . . . I'll return to normal . . . right?"

"Oh, Mrs. Harriss," Dr. Morlen informed me, "you will most likely need to remain in isolation, possibly for the rest of your life, even if it's in your own home."

Terrified, I turned to Mom. As she hugged me I remembered talking to some patients in the waiting room who had not left their homes in years except to make their occasional journey to the clinic. My mind could not even begin to fathom how horrible that would be. I suddenly realized I was in a fight for my life.

CHAPTER TWO

ABANDONED AND ALONE

But if I go to the east, he is not there; if I go to the west,
I do not find him.
—Job 23:8

IN SPITE OF DR. MORLEN'S INSISTENCE, I refused to be admitted into the hospital. Somehow, I was determined to overcome this breakdown in my body like I had tackled every other obstacle in my life—on my own.

Dr. Morlen advised me that we would have to make major changes in our home if I insisted on living there. It was imperative that we seal off the doors to the new game room.

The toxic chemicals in the building materials would completely destroy my immune system if I continued to breathe the fumes. We needed to remove all the carpeting, drapes, rugs, and wall decorations throughout the house. Our gas appliances, anything with an odor or scent, had to be eliminated. He advised us to eliminate household dust as much as possible. In other words, we were to strip out our entire home.

Life Turned Upside Down

My bedroom would have to be converted into an isolation unit, with bed and bedding replaced with an aluminum cot and cotton quilts for a mattress.

"You'll need to keep an oxygen tank beside your cot at all times," Dr. Morlen added.

"What?" I cried. "Why?"

"The oxygen will help reduce the swelling in your brain and, therefore, the pain throughout your body when you have allergic reactions to food or chemical exposures."

"I hardly see how that can happen if I follow all your other instructions." I couldn't keep a touch of frustration from creeping into my voice.

"Even if you do everything you are supposed to, if someone comes into your room wearing anything with chemicals—new shoes, clothing, hair spray, colognes . . ."

"I get the picture," I groaned.

"You will also need the oxygen on days when pollens in the air are high, or if it rains."

"Don't tell me I'm allergic to rain!"

"Moisture in the air and ground elevates the mold count."

"Great." Mold had been a major disaster for me during testing.

"You won't be able to use a standard oxygen mask, because they're made of plastic."

By now I was skeptical. *What am I, a freak? How can anyone be allergic to plastic? Everything in the world is made out of plastic!*

"We'll have to get you a specially designed ceramic mask."

I couldn't imagine living like this. "Anything else?" I asked with a sense of despair.

"You'll also have to remove all reading materials," Dr. Morlen informed me. "Books, magazines, newspapers . . ."

"You can't be serious," I groaned. Reading would help to pass my time away if I was going to live in isolation. "I have to at least be able to read my Bible!" I decided no matter how my body reacted, I refused to give up my time in God's Word. Nothing was more important to me. It was my lifeline, but I was allergic to the formaldehyde on the paper, the mold that formed on the paper, and the ink used for printing.

"The only way you can read is by using this." Dr. Morlen showed me an 18" by 24" box made of stainless steel and glass. The glass slid to one end so reading material could be inserted. I turned it over in my hands. There were openings on the sides with cotton gloves attached. Apparently, I was supposed to turn pages by slipping my hands into the box through the gloves.

"How do the books and magazines get in there in the first place if I'm not supposed to touch them?" I asked.

"Your friends or family members will have to place them into the box for you."

It was surreal. *If I stare out this window long enough, will I eventually wake up from this nightmare?* I set the heavy box on his desk. "Doctor Morlen, you don't understand. I can't rely on other people to do everything for me. I'm much too independent to live like that."

"No, Linda," Dr. Morlen corrected, "You don't understand. This is the only way you can possibly survive and get somewhat better. You must create as pure an environment as possible because you will spend your time in that room."

My mind tried to comprehend what he was telling me. "What do you mean?"

"As long as your immune system is functioning so poorly," he explained, "you must spend twenty-four hours a day, seven days a week, in an environment as completely pure as possible."

"Isn't there anything you can do for me?" I asked in desperation.

"Of course," he said. I wondered if he really believed there was hope for me or if this was the response doctors were trained to give to all of their hopeless cases. "Your new diet, which will consist of all organic foods, will hopefully help a lot."

Peggy, the nutritionist, had provided me with a special diet plan consisting solely of green beans, carrots, avocados, almonds, apples, and chicken. The chicken would have to be baked, the vegetables cooked in a small amount of boiling spring water. I could use no seasonings other than salt, and no butter or oil of any kind. The only liquid I could drink was spring water because tap water contained chlorine—yet another substance I was severely allergic to.

"Great," I said without enthusiasm. "Anything else?"

"Well," he said slowly, apparently trying to come up with something to placate me. "Allergy shots may also help."

Great. I love shots. As a nurse, I didn't mind giving them. But I hated being on the receiving end. "Do I really need injections?" I asked with a wince.

"They will allow you to better tolerate your food and environment," Dr. Morlen explained patiently. "They may even neutralize some of your allergic reactions. They should also help reduce your pain throughout your entire body," he added.

"Can't I just take a good pain reliever when I need to?" I asked. "Aspirin? Tylenol?"

"Those remedies might be more effective in controlling pain than the injections," Dr. Morlen conceded. "Unfortunately, you are allergic to both of them."

That figures!

"You will have to teach your husband how to administer your injections." Dr. Morlen informed me.

"You're kidding," I said. "Earl hates shots more than I do."

"You'll have to receive eight per day, every single day," Dr. Morlen explained. "Two at 8 a.m., two more at noon, two at 4, and the last two at 8 p.m. Each injection will contain several allergens, the number varying, depending on how badly you react to the things around you. If you are having a lot of reactions, you will have serotonin to relieve your symptoms. Your dosage has been calculated and written on the vial."

"Is all that really necessary?" I asked.

"Yes." Dr. Morlen's eyes bored into mine. "If you want to go on living."

I took a deep breath that did little to calm my quivering nerves. "Do you think I will ever function normally again?" I asked around a lump in my throat.

"I can't really answer that question, Linda," he said with a sigh. "Your immune system has been extremely damaged." His eyes were filled with compassion. I would have preferred they be filled with optimism. "The situation doesn't look hopeful at this point. Your one chance is to follow my instructions implicitly. That's the only way for you to avoid further chemical exposure."

"And what will happen if I experience further chemical exposure?" The thought of being isolated in my room was terrifying. *Could the alternatives be so horrible that isolation was the better choice?*

Dr. Morlen responded with painful honesty. "It would continue to damage your immune system further, leaving your body predisposed to any number of traumatic diseases, or even death."

I had never felt so completely overwhelmed. My mind as foggy as it was most of the time, I tried to comprehend all that Dr. Morlen was saying.

Grappling with Reality

I cried all the way home on our six-hour drive from the doctor's office, staring at the new diet clutched in my trembling hands. I still couldn't believe what I had been told and wanted to start running and not stop. I never wanted to face the world again.

"Why has this happened?" I asked my mother over and over.

Her reply was always the same. "Baby, I just don't know."

"But this is so unfair," I cried. "Not just to me, but to our whole family. We've all worked so hard to build and furnish our home, and now we're supposed to just tear it all apart?" I trembled with sadness and confusion. "I won't do it," I determined. I refused to give in to this crazy illness.

"Let's just pray for the Lord to lead us," Mom replied.

Early in life Mom taught me by her words and example that in every situation we could trust God. While I was someone who wanted everything to be explained and proven, her faith was basic and simple. She loved and trusted Jesus more than life itself. So many times in the midst of life's storms,

Mom didn't consider the circumstances around her, but stood on an un-shakable faith that never wavered. That had always seemed so simplistic to me, but now it comforted me. I looked at Mom with tears running down my cheeks. Without her speaking a word, I knew she would be standing in the gap praying and believing for me like she had always done before.

Nobody hated being sick more than I did. I resented having to depend on others to take care of me. I was supposed to take care of everyone else. That was what I was trained to do.

My greatest concern was how to tell my children that I could no longer be part of their world because their world made me deathly ill. They would never understand. What could they say to their friends? They would be so troubled by my crazy situation.

An internal battle was raging in more ways than one. I had no peace. Fear was beginning to consume me. Hopelessness and despair were my con-stant companions. For the first time in my life, I was feeling powerless and that I had no purpose. Still . . . I was not willing to succumb to defeat. My personality resonated, pushing me to do everything, do it now, and rely on my life-long training that always seemed to get me the results I wanted. I was fiercely determined to persevere and make things happen. Besides, my iden-tity and sense of self were tied to what I could accomplish and do for others.

When we got home, I started looking at everything in my house that caused me tremendous pain and depression. Our home, which had long been a source of love and happiness, was now nothing more than a death trap.

I made my decision. I would adhere to the unbelievably strict diet and suffer through the shots. I would have the braces taken off my teeth. I even consented to restricting my out-of-home activities, since I did not have con-trol over the outside environment or other people. But I adamantly refused to completely isolate myself from my family and decided I would not stay in my room. I wouldn't seal off the game room and would continue to wear my ordinary clothes. I wouldn't create a safe room, and I'd keep going to activities away from home that I felt were safe for me.

I had always been strong and determined, and saw no reason to stop now, believing that my own strength and persistence could keep me going when the medical experts were telling me to give in. I would do what I felt I could, for there was no way I was going to just roll over and give up. As a nurse, I'd seen patients just give up and passively accept what was happening to them. I was not going to be that patient.

Besides, I had my strong faith in God on my side; I was determined to overcome this with His help. I thought that if I just trusted Him enough, He would be all that I needed.

Faith Tested

Much to Earl's dismay, he learned how to administer my injections and became quite good at it. The children quickly bestowed on him the title, "Dr. Harriss."

Unfortunately, I almost always had an adverse reaction to the shots.

I started calling some of my Christian friends to seek their advice on how I should handle this bizarre illness. The consensus seemed to be that if I had enough faith, confessed my sins, and claimed healing, I would receive it. That sounded great! If all it took was for me to muster up enough faith to escape this horrible illness, then I would do whatever was required to get it. Besides, walking in faith sounded like an easy choice compared to making all the changes Dr. Morlen recommended.

I began claiming every healing Scripture in the Bible. I prayed for more faith. I made positive statements. "Thank you, Lord, I am healed," I practically chanted. But I continued to grow worse. Never had I felt like such a failure in my Christian life. At times I would get discouraged and would begin to question my every belief about God and my salvation. I became confused and angry with God, even doubting if He existed at all.

Then I would be consumed with guilt as those thoughts raced through my mind. I knew there was a God, but at times I felt so abandoned and alone. I had to work hard to keep focused on God's Truth rather than the irrational thoughts and emotions that ran through my mind.

Why were non-Christians sometimes healed, yet I couldn't conjure up enough faith to bring healing in my own life? I just didn't understand. After all, I had been a Christian since age 11!

Anger welled up inside me. I still couldn't believe this was happening! I loved life and my family. I had always been quite active in the church and community. I really enjoyed occasionally filling in at the hospital and my job as a school nurse. Through my confusion and feelings of failure, I went straight to the Word. I sought truth like I had never sought it before.

A Spiritual Roller Coaster

Still, my depression grew deeper—right out of the pits of hell. I didn't think I could take it much longer. Even some of the foods I was least allergic to caused severe allergic reactions, as did everything in my environment. Never in my life had I felt so mistreated and unloved by God. But He continued to speak to my spirit, assuring me that He loved me.

Satan, on the other hand, put doubts in my mind. "If God really loved you," he seemed to whisper in my ear, "you would already be healed." I knew I was in the middle of a spiritual tug of war, but was determined to respond to this disease according to my faith despite the roller coaster of emotions, doubts and fears.

I began talking to Christians who were open to God's healing in ways I'd not known before. Some were more helpful than others. In fact, a few claimed my health was a result of unconfessed sin or lack of belief or spiritual weakness, which compelled me to address any hidden faults and scour the Bible for passages on healing. Despite this, I was still afflicted. Once in desperation I even called the 800 number on the screen of a televised Christian program. I called another TV program and made the obligatory positive statements. "Thank you, Lord, I am healed," I said repeatedly.

The advice didn't stop there. A few of my well-intentioned Christian acquaintances advised me to quit taking the shots. And, I wanted to stop the shots. Every fiber of my being wanted to forget the whole business. But

I knew I couldn't go that far. According to the doctor, my very life depended on those shots. I was in a dilemma, because I longed to be healed, but my body didn't seem to want to go along with my plans. So I continued to grow worse, caught in a tormented mix of facts and fear and faith . . . and failure.

Honestly, at times I would get discouraged and would begin to question my every belief about God and my salvation. I became more and more confused and angry with God, even doubting if He existed at all. Again, I would be consumed with waves of guilt as those thoughts raced through my mind. But throughout the confusion, deep within my heart and soul, I knew God loved me and I had to trust Him rather than my roller coaster emotions.

Challenges of Summer

Summertime in Texas is always extremely hot, and 1985 was certainly no exception. The heat was unbearable. We usually ran the air conditioner all summer long, using the natural-gas wells on our property. But Dr. Morlen had advised me that the gas air conditioner was one of the things I could possibly be reacting to. We couldn't believe this was true, so we ignored his advice and ran it anyway.

One day the temperature reached 101 degrees outside, and the house felt even hotter. Mom went to the hall to check the setting on the thermostat. The dial was set properly, but the unit wasn't running. Earl went outside to check the regulator, thinking the gas pressure might be too low. The meter showed sufficient output, but for some unexplainable reason the air-conditioning unit had simply shut off. He tried to reset it, but without success. So Earl went to the gas well in the field. Everything seemed fine. Puzzled, he returned to the house and reset the regulator. This time, the unit started running and the house began to cool. But a few hours later, it shut off again. This cycle recurred several times. In fact, the next day was a rerun of the day before. Earl performed all the same checks and could find no apparent reason for the air conditioner to shut off.

"Earl," I finally said, "maybe the Lord is trying to show us something. Perhaps the gas running the unit really is making me sick."

"I'm going to try something else," he said and headed out the door. Still unsure of what was happening, he drove into town and bought a new regulator. As soon as it was installed, the house began to cool. We all cheered. But the following day the unit shut off again for no apparent reason.

Finally Earl shook his head and said, "Babe, you're right. God must be trying to tell us not to run the air conditioner."

We decided to change out all the gas appliances for electric ones—the oven, the cooktop, water heaters, cooling and heating systems. Both the air-conditioning unit and the gas water heater were new, and each had cost hundreds of dollars. Having just spent so much on my medical expenses, we really couldn't afford this. But we believed the Lord had spoken through these occurrences, so the changes were made.

The days grew hotter. My son, Greg, played in the community summer baseball league, and I was determined not to miss his games. But the dust and cigarette smoke in the bleachers were more than I could tolerate, so Earl came up with a plan. He drove his truck to the ballpark early, parking it right up close to the fence. Then his mother took me in my car—Earl had thoroughly vacuumed and washed all the dash and trim with baking soda to neutralize any chemical smells. He had meticulously cleaned his mother's car, as well. She drove me to the ballpark, where we slipped into the spot Earl had secured. He re-parked the truck and then split his time between sitting in the car with me and standing close to the dugout to encourage Greg.

The temperature reached 103 degrees that day, but the car windows had to stay rolled up tight to keep out the environment. Hot tears poured down my cheeks. I held a large bowl of ice water in my lap and cooled my face and neck with wet washcloths. Earl and his mom did the same. How I wanted to be sitting outside in those stands, cheering and supporting Greg like I had done for years.

Besides the normal pollens and dust in the air, the ballpark was close to the industrial area where several large manufacturing plants were located. Frequently the area was filled with strong, toxic chemical odors that were released from the factories. Not only were the baseball field and surrounding areas filled with the smell of chemicals, but those same toxic fumes reached our house several miles away when the wind reached our house. There were days when the smell of chemicals was so bad that I didn't want Greg and Christie outside.

Frustrated, I contacted the EPA to test the air emitted from one of the plants. They did so, but unfortunately they came on a weekend when the factory was not releasing the toxins into the air. As a result, I was informed the chemicals emitted into the atmosphere were within acceptable guidelines, and the air was considered to be safe for humans to breathe. I confronted the EPA representative when he visited my house, asking why the testing was done on a day when the plant was not releasing the pollutants. I asked him if management at the plant knew when the testing would be done. He informed me that by law, the EPA had to tell the plant when the testing would take place. I didn't agree with their manner of testing nor the reports presented to me. But at the time I didn't have the energy to fight them.

Family, Friends and Coping

My condition grew worse. The children became depressed. Their summer days, which should have been filled with fun and happy hours, were instead full of worry, sadness, and tears. Greg, who was in seventh grade, spent an inordinate amount of time in his room working on his coin and baseball-card collections, obviously trying to distract himself from dealing with my illness. More than once I saw Christie, who was in ninth grade, lying across her bed, staring at the walls and crying. My sense of guilt for their pain and despair swallowed me up.

I couldn't stand it. I felt so guilty. Just knowing my children were hurting because of me was more than I could handle. Our family had always been so happy. Now it was a nightmare that seemed would never end. How could this be happening to us?

July came, and most of my days were spent in bed, buried in deep depression. At times I just wanted to give up and die. I was embarrassed, feeling misunderstood, feeling different, feeling alone.

Little did I realize the depths of this spiritual warfare. I felt I was battling for my heart and soul. Desiring to stand strong in my journey of faith and being so drained from the fighting, many times I just wanted to surrender and let life take its course. But something deep within me kept me from giving up.

One day, as I rested while watching television—with Earl's mother, whom we called Grandmother, sleeping in the bed next to me—a Christian program came on. I was in a great deal of physical pain and wasn't really listening to what the evangelist was saying. But something caught my attention when he began speaking about God's healing powers. Suddenly, my whole body started to light-up. I saw my skin and clothes glowing as if my whole body were illuminated. I realized that something supernatural was happening to me.

I wanted to ask Grandmother to look at me and see what was happening. But when I tried to turn my head, I realized I was unable to speak or even move. As I lay there wanting desperately to speak to her, I finally became aware that I had to relinquish control of my body in total submission to a Power much higher than myself. I knew without a doubt that this Power was Almighty God revealing Himself to me in a new way, unlike anything I had ever experienced before. The illumination and immobilization lasted about thirty seconds. When I was finally able to move again, I was so excited I could hardly wait to wake up Grandmother and tell her what had happened.

As I was about to touch her shoulder, I hesitated. What if I had just imagined everything? I'd always considered miraculous signs and wonders to be events that took place typically only during Biblical days. Though the doubt was tempting, I also knew I couldn't give in to it and had to embrace the occurrence as a sign from God that He was at work in my life.

Still unsure of what to say to Grandmother, I gently woke her. But before I could say a word, she quickly began describing a dream she'd just had about me. "I was walking down the dirt road that runs through the fields on our farm," she said. "As I looked ahead I saw something lying in the road. It was glowing so brightly it almost blinded me. When I walked over to it, I saw it was a fish. I bent over to pick it up, but a voice said, 'Don't touch that. It's part of Linda's healing.' So I just stood there, staring at the fish. It was still glowing—like it was illuminated."

I was baffled as to the significance of the fish. But her use of the word illuminated held great meaning for me, because that's how my body had looked when I couldn't move. I knew the Lord was confirming to me, and to her, that I was going to be healed.

At times, momentarily, deep down, I was still uneasy. I began to question what had taken place. Whenever I heard people give accounts of miracles, visions, and hearing audibly from the Lord, I sometimes considered them nothing more than emotional experiences or exaggerations. This experience certainly wasn't emotional—it was supernatural. God was revealing Himself to me as never before.

At times the enemy would try to make me believe; that surely these things were just coincidental or brought about by my intense desires for healing. But as skeptical as I tried to be—as intense as the spiritual warfare was—I could not deny the sense of hope and belief that had begun to glimmer in my soul.

All summer I'd been claiming healing and confessing sin and asking for prayer—and all of that was me trying very hard to make something happen. But none of those efforts caused the kind of hope and belief that this had. Something different had happened, something that I couldn't cause by my own effort. I began to understand that the Lord can give us spiritual eyes and spiritual ears for us to see and hear what He has for us. Scripture gives accounts of God speaking through dreams, visions, signs, and wonders. Before long I would understand the significance of my experience and Grandmother's dream of the "illuminated" fish.

I refused to look in a mirror. It frightened me to see my life wasting away before my eyes, and barely could recognize myself. On occasions when I had visitors, they didn't know what to say. I was so thin, my pale skin was stretched taut over my entire frame. Every bone of my body pressed an outline like a morbid relief map of my skeleton. I had always enjoyed my long, thick, shiny hair. But when I got sick, it became dull and I lost half of it. I worried that I would need to wear a wig. Then I realized I wouldn't be able to wear wigs because of the synthetic materials used to make them.

I had dedicated my entire adult life to being a wife and mother, and now I couldn't fill either role. Not only could I not be there for my children and husband, but for the past four months I couldn't be there for anyone. None of this fazed Earl. He planned our future when I only saw death. Besides being severely ill and physically weak, I was constantly in a state of depression. I struggled daily with guilt about this.

I still couldn't fathom how foods, air-borne inhalants, and chemicals could cause such severe depression. I could understand these things causing skin rashes, headaches, stuffed up noses, shortness of breath, etc. But I had cerebral reactions. My brain re-wired when exposed to these things, resulting in this beneath the pits of hell depression and numerous other bizarre complications. I felt totally incapacitated, leaving me drowning in shame. I was failing in my attempt to "get through this" and get back to life.

Fortunately, it lifted my spirits and momentarily eased my anguish and depression every time people called or came to visit me (if they weren't wearing something that caused me to react). The emotional chaos that whirled constantly throughout my mind was temporarily stilled, giving me a short respite from the agony and misery.

 Per Dr. Morlen's instructions, whenever someone wanted to visit me, I informed them of all the necessary prerequisites. All my visitors had to wash their hair in unscented shampoo. Wearing new or recently dry-cleaned clothes was not allowed because of the strong chemical smells that were emitted. They could wear no perfume, cologne, aftershave, hair spray, lotion, or makeup. They could not even be chewing gum or mints. Purses and shoes had to be left outside my room.

I hated creating hassles for everyone around me. But it seemed every time someone came to visit me, my body reacted to something they were wearing. When my friends started to realize this, most of them simply stopped coming. They did not want to make me sick. Besides, I knew it was unreasonable to ask people to take all the strange and inconvenient precautions necessary just so I wouldn't become ill.

I felt abandoned by almost everyone, including God. I needed someone to "stand in the gap" for me. To believe for me. To pray for me. To praise God for me.

One hot summer day, as I rested in my room feeling particularly lonely and isolated, I heard sweet voices filtering in through my bedroom window. With great effort, I pulled myself out of bed and peeked outside. There in the yard stood several of my dearest friends: Pam Erikson, Kathy Rodgers, Mrs. Lindsey, Sherry Tunnel, and even Betty Wilson, a friend from church who was battling cancer.

They sang beautiful praise songs for me out there on my lawn. Betty played the accordion and Pam accompanied her on a tambourine. They sang "Let's Just Praise the Lord" and then "I Will Enter His Gates." Tears streamed down my face. I felt so unworthy of such special friends. I was overcome with emotion, especially seeing Betty singing and praising God in her cancer-weakened state. Never had I been so ministered to by a group of friends. I literally felt as if I was in the presence of Almighty God and His heavenly hosts. I was so grateful for their visit even if it was from outside the bedroom window. I felt so validated and loved.

Hospital on the Horizon

As the summer progressed, my symptoms grew worse. One Sunday as I sat in my bedroom praying, Earl came in and said he'd been on the front porch praying.

"Babe," he announced, "I think you need to go to the hospital for further evaluation, like Dr. Morlen recommended."

Deep in my spirit I knew he was right. But I had been battling so desperately to claim my healing by faith. I sought advice from Christian friends, dug deep into the crevices of my mind, and confessed my sins—even those that I wasn't really for sure that I had committed. I called into Christian TV programs and requested prayer, hoping the people answering the phones had greater power in their prayers than I had in mine. I looked up every healing scripture in the Bible and tried to memorize them. I made positive statements that I was healed. Nothing seemed to work. I never liked to wait to get things done and was accustomed to immediate results for my efforts.

I had always been very disciplined and strong in my belief. But now I felt so badly physically and mentally that I was confused beyond any ability to make a reasonable decision. One of my ongoing allergic reactions was mental fogginess. We discussed this momentous step of going to the hospital for a while, then finally gave up on making a decision.

A few minutes later, the telephone rang. "Hello, Linda, this is Mrs. McMillan. I don't know if you remember me, but I met you once a long time ago."

I remembered her, but only vaguely.

"Our Sunday school class prayed for you this morning, and as we prayed, the Holy Spirit spoke to me quite clearly."

I was hesitant to hear what she had to say because so many people had already told me what God would have me do. Some told me to stop taking the shots. Others told me to just ignore the symptoms . . . how could I ignore my body shutting down? Mostly I was told that I just needed more faith. Their suggestions were given with good intent, but I just wanted to hear from Him directly.

"The Spirit told me," she continued, "not to stay after Sunday school for the church service, but to go straight home and call you. The Lord led me to tell you about a group of doctors in Houston who are terrific in treating allergies."

Just what I need—a bunch of doctors to run a slew of tests and tell me that nothing can be done for my condition.

But Mrs. McMillan's next words made me sit upright on my bed. "There is a clinic in Houston that specializes in severe allergies. They also have a special unit in a hospital for patients with Environmental Illness."

When I told Earl about the phone call, we knew without a doubt that the Lord had used Mrs. McMillan to confirm His will for me to go into the hospital that Dr. Morlen had earlier recommended. We now realized that the Lord had been telling us to do this all along. But we had chosen not to follow His plan because we thought it would show a lack of faith. We chose to believe that if I just had enough faith I could be healed. As a result I had only grown worse.

This time we didn't hesitate. Bright and early the next morning Earl made the arrangements for me to be checked into the hospital. It felt like a defeat in a way, and it was. I was having to let go of just a bit of my determination to fix things my own way in my own strength. I had no idea how strong that battle was going to be. Giving up the idea that I could manage my own life was to be as big a battle as the battle against my illness.

The thought of leaving my home and family was terrifying. But we knew we had heard from the Lord, so two days later we said our good-byes to our children and parents through tear-filled eyes and soon were on our way.

CHAPTER THREE

NO LONGER A PART OF THE REAL WORLD

Keep me safe, O God, for in you I take refuge.
—Psalm 16:1

WITH GREAT HESITATION, on Tuesday, August 6, 1985, we got in our vehicle and made the long trip to Houston. As Earl drove into the hospital parking lot, my heart began to race, almost pounding out of my chest. When he parked, I inched to the edge of the seat and slowly got out. Standing beside the car, I suddenly felt an overwhelming urge to start running, but wasn't sure where I could go to escape this horrible situation. As my thoughts raced out of control, Psalm 55:6-7 flashed through my mind: "Oh, that I had wings like a dove! I would fly away and be at rest. Indeed, I would wander far off, and remain in the wilderness" (NKJV).

Earl sensed my fear and walked to my side, pulling me close and hugging me for several minutes. Then he took my hand and slowly led me to the entrance of the hospital. As we walked together, hands clutched tightly, I faced my new reality for the first time. No longer could I pretend or deny the seriousness of my illness. Feeling totally overwhelmed, yet fighting to be brave, I brushed the tears off my cheeks. Earl's eyes were filled with tears, as well. Surely he had a lot of the same fears and concerns that I had. I was so blessed to have such a wonderfully committed husband. I felt so undeserving of his love and was so grateful for him.

As we approached the entrance, I stopped and just stood there, staring at the huge doors. I knew that once I went through them my life would forever be changed. *Lord, you are my only hope and strength. Please don't leave me.*

Reluctantly, I was admitted to the Environmentally Controlled Unit of the Houston Hospital for three to four weeks of allergy testing. Very likely I faced another month or two to stabilize my condition, which was terrifying. I certainly didn't want to be away from Earl, who had always protected me and kept me safe. But we didn't have much of a choice. It seemed my body was trying to shut down, for no matter what I ate, drank or smelled, I had severe reactions. It felt as though I was fighting the whole world trying to survive.

Never had I felt so helpless, weak, and without hope.

A Sterile New World

The lady at the information center in the lobby directed us. "Take those elevators up to the fourth floor. The ward for Universal Reactors is at the end of the hall."

I hated to hear those words—Universal Reactors. The last thing I wanted was to admit that I was a part of such a strange group. Feelings of embarrassment crowded out all other emotions. I hated that no one understood what I was going through. I had never before felt like an outsider, but now found myself in a group of people that I certainly didn't want to be a part of.

Once inside the elevator, though, I was again haunted by fear. As the doors reopened, I saw a sign that pointed to the Environmentally Controlled Unit. Stepping out into the corridor, my heart began to race even faster. My grip on Earl's hand tightened.

Why can't I wake up from this nightmare? This can't really be happening to me. Lord, are you there?

We finally reached a set of big metal doors and entered. A nurse smiled as we approached the glass-enclosed front desk. She was the only sign of life I saw in the room.

"Hi. My name is Carolyn," she said in a soft, kind voice. "I'll be your nurse today." Carolyn was petite, with dark brown hair and eyes. Although she was very pretty, she wore no makeup—undoubtedly because of the patients' allergies to chemicals and scents. "You've been assigned to room 449B," she said. "But first let me give you a tour of the facility."

Carolyn led us down a long, dim hallway. "The walls here are painted with a non-toxic, odorless, no VOC (Volatile Organic Compounds) paint," she explained. "Some are covered with ceramic tiles with non-toxic grout. The flooring is tile since carpets are a major source of toxic pollutants and harbor dust and molds." She opened a door marked Suite 405. "Our offices," she informed us, "have been designed to eliminate all obvious sources of offending substances. The walls and cabinets are created from baked porcelain over steel."

Carolyn stopped in front of a row of desks. "Computers and printers outgas low levels of toxic emissions into the air," she pointed out, "so we have encased the backs and sides in stainless steel boxes. Those cases vent the machines into special filtration devices, which minimizes air contamination."

Next, we were led past a row of examination rooms. "The testing-room chairs are made of metal with hard plastic seats. The hard plastic material doesn't outgas toxins like softer plastics. All of our wood furniture has been specially constructed for us, using high-grade white oak, created and hand-carved in a special low-contamination shop using modified equipment," she explained. "The cushions on the furniture and the pillows on the examination-room tables are made with hand-loomed, organically grown cotton fabric that was developed using color-grown, not dyed, fibers. The stuffing is also made of natural cotton."

I noticed all the exam-room tables were metal. They looked cold—as cold and uninviting as the rest of this place.

"A large central air system is employed throughout the clinic," Carolyn said, continuing our tour, "with special devices designed for air filtration. These units are made from stainless steel and have four types of filters: a pre-filter of aluminum mesh, coconut charcoal, paper—with no glues, of course—and glass beads. These remove not only pollens, dust, and molds, but also the chemicals that many standard air filters do not."

What a lot of hard work and effort, I thought, *just so people can breathe.*

"The water throughout the clinic is filtered to remove biological and chemical contaminants. The specially designed filters contain no plastic parts, leaving the water in a highly purified state."

When did air and water become such complex commodities? I wondered in silence.

"Naturally," she added, "the ward is entirely pesticide free."

I looked up at Earl, wondering if he could read my thoughts. Without pesticides, I wondered how they handled insects. But I didn't care enough to ask. I just wanted this tour, and the rest of my stay here, to be over as quickly as possible.

"Here we are," Carolyn finally said. "Room 449B." She pushed open the metal door.

A Room for Two

The room looked like an empty bank vault. The walls were all stainless steel, the floor a subdued gray ceramic tile. No decorations of any kind graced the walls or tables. Unlike most hospital rooms, no cheery bouquets of flowers, balloons, or stuffed animals were allowed here. All the lights were covered with strange filters that made the place seem dim and frightening.

"This is your roommate, Flo," Carolyn introduced, pointing to an elderly lady lying on one of the beds. "She's from Ohio."

Contorted and twisted, Flo's body was obviously ravaged with pain. Strange pieces of equipment surrounded her. A heart monitor was hooked up to her chest. She received oxygen through a tube, and blood via an IV needle in her arm.

I panicked. *Please, God, don't make me stay in here with her!*

"Flo is bedfast," Carolyn explained. "She's too critical to do much of anything for herself."

"Shouldn't she be in the Intensive Care Unit?" I asked.

"This hospital doesn't have an ICU for Environmentally Ill patients," Carolyn explained, reminding me again that I was not one of the normal people. "Even the critical ones stay here with the other patients."

I asked Carolyn to step out into the hall with me.

"Please," I begged, "can I get a different room?" I was thinking that I wouldn't be comfortable being in a room with someone who was so ill. My mind was racing and my heart was pounding. Was there something that Dr. Morlen hadn't told me? Looking at Flo, seeing her lifeless emaciated body, I asked myself, *Am I looking at myself in the near future?* I didn't want a constant reminder of how ill I really was.

She hesitated, looking at me like I was a finicky patron in a posh resort hotel. "Let me check on availability," she finally said.

As Earl and I waited, still holding hands, I was suddenly overcome with a sense that I had not been assigned to this room by accident. I felt God had specifically placed this frail little person in my life for me to minister to, in spite of the fact that I could barely care for myself.

I tugged on Earl's hand. As he turned to look at me, I whispered, "Babe, I feel like I should stay here with Flo after all."

His protective nature kicked in. "I don't want you to stay in a room with anyone if it's going to stress you out or make you sad."

"I think it will be all right," I explained. "I believe the Lord has ordained that I be in this room."

Earl agreed with my decision to stay. Still not happy with the thought, but resigned to the fact that this was apparently what I was supposed to do, I walked out of the room and down the hall to find Carolyn.

"I'll stay with Flo in 449B," I said. She looked at me in obvious surprise. I did not even begin to explain my reasons. How could I? I was more confused than she! So Carolyn walked us back down the hall. This time, I peeked into some of the rooms along the way.

This place, these people—they don't belong to the real world. Everyone looked thin, pale, and emaciated. Death seemed to hover in every corner. I didn't want to be a part of their world, but there did not seem to be an escape. *Can you hear me, God? Do you have an escape for me?*

No one was dressed like a normal person. Everyone wore white pajamas. "They're made of 100 percent organic cotton, custom made for and furnished by the hospital," Carolyn explained as we reached 449B and she handed me my own set of prison garb. "The patients here can't wear street clothes because the dyes and chemicals in synthetic fabrics cause severe reactions."

So that's why I passed out in the new clothing store in town!

"The laundry is washed in a natural, chemical-free soap, then rinsed in baking soda." Carolyn directed me to the bathroom adjoining my room. "We have special hairbrushes and toothbrushes made of natural materials. No toothpaste is allowed here—you'll use baking soda instead. The soap for bathing and hair washing has been specially ordered without chemicals or scent. No makeup or perfumes, of course." I wasn't even allowed to use my electric hair rollers because they were made of plastic. When heated, they released smells of plastic and chemicals into the atmosphere.

It seemed the world was filled with invisible toxins lurking in innocent, everyday places, just waiting to strike with their deadly venom. No wonder the people of the world are so plagued with cancer and other diseases.

I didn't want to think about this anymore. It was too overwhelming and frightening, more than anyone could possibly be expected to understand. I felt like the world was spinning by, but couldn't grab hold of it.

Carolyn left the room and I put on my prison uniform. Then I slumped on the bed and stared at the wall. I couldn't face Earl because I was fighting so hard to hold back the tears. We were both too emotional to talk. We sat there quietly trying to comprehend everything around us. Flo just lay there, staring out the window. The only sounds in the room were the rattles and wheezes of her monitoring equipment.

An Eventful Lunch

Finally, Carolyn came in with lunch. My tray had nothing on it but a small mound of baked yellow squash. "Due to the severity of your food allergies," Carolyn explained, "and in order to reduce the intensity of your reactions, Dr. Morlen has restricted your diet to only one food at a time."

I looked down at my plate, then back up at Carolyn. She had placed a second tray at Flo's bedside and removed the lid. Soon she was spooning pureed mush into the elderly woman's mouth. "Turkey and carrots today, Flo," she said with a smile. I stared at my plate of squash. At least I wasn't too weak to chew my own food.

Carolyn poured another spoonful of pureed food into Flo's mouth, scooping a little off the old woman's lower lip. "You'd better eat up," Carolyn urged me. "Doctor's orders say you're supposed to start fasting at midnight tonight."

At Earl's nod of encouragement, I started picking at the tiny, bland meal. Would it make me ill, like everything else I'd tried to eat in recent months? Even if it did, what choice did I have? It's difficult to decide between symptoms and starvation.

"Is that all you can eat today, Flo?" Carolyn asked my ailing roommate. "That's all right, you just get some rest now." She drew the curtain between our beds, then left with Flo's tray, promising to return later for mine. Before I had taken more than a few bites, a tall, slender nurse came into the room. "Hello, Linda," she said, placing a hand on my shoulder. "I'm Peggy, your nutritional consultant. I'll be working with you to try to find foods that you are best able to tolerate."

Sounds good to me, I thought as I stared at the yellow mush on my plate.

"According to your health history, you've lost twenty-two pounds over the last few months, which has left you considerably underweight and malnourished. It is vital that we get accurate results of the food-allergy testing so I can plan your diet each day."

I hated this illness. Not only was I unable to prepare meals for my family, I was apparently incapable of planning my own.

"We'll need to detox your system before we can start the allergy testing," Peggy explained. "We have to make sure it's completely clear in order to achieve more accurate test results. I'm afraid you'll have to fast for the next four days."

"That'll be easy," I shrugged. I'd basically been starving for months. What were four more days?

Peggy explained that she would be monitoring my weight as well as the status of my fat and muscle mass so she could accurately assess my health. She placed calipers on my waist and underarms, recording the measurements on a form attached to her clipboard. According to her results I had very little muscle or fat mass left on my body.

God, do you know what it is like for your whole body to turn against you? Do you know my pain? Forgive me. Of course you do. Jesus was beaten, tortured, and humiliated, and then hung on a cross to die. You certainly didn't deserve what happened to you, either.

Peggy studied the results, then shook her head and stared at me. "I honestly don't know where to begin to help you," she said with a sigh. "But I will do my best."

That was certainly comforting. I looked at Earl for reassurance, like I always did whenever I was frightened about something.

"Babe, don't worry," he said. "You're going to be all right. I will never stop praying for you and believing that God will bring you through this."

I wondered what Flo must be thinking about our conversation. With the curtain drawn between my bed and hers, I was unable to see her response.

After Peggy left, Carolyn came back in. "I want you to sign this consent form," she said.

"What's this for?" I asked absently, beyond really caring what they wanted to do to me next.

"It's for a consultation with a psychologist," she explained.

My pen stopped in midair and I peered into Carolyn's eyes. "What?"

"The psychologist can help you learn to cope with your illness."

"That will not be necessary," I said firmly, refusing to sign. "I don't need to talk to anyone about my situation." I preferred to pretend it didn't exist. Besides, I came from a family who does not admit to or discuss problems in our lives. We just handle them. *Lord, you are the Great Physician. If I sign this, it will look like I'm not trusting you, like I have a lack of faith. Please strengthen my faith according to 2 Timothy 2:13, "If we are faithless, he remains faithful."*

Earl added his authoritative response. "Linda doesn't need a psychologist. We can handle this situation just fine once she gets the medical help she needs."

Carolyn shook her head and left with the unsigned papers and my lunch tray.

Flo and Friends

My stubborn, independent mindset didn't allow me to accept the wisdom and guidance that a psychologist could give me. I had never been given permission to ask for help . . . the very thing that I needed to survive this life threatening ordeal—psychological help. *What would people think if I was counseled? Would they think I was crazy? Would I be giving up my independence? Would it appear that I had a lack of faith? Besides people trained to be psychologist and counselors probably don't focus on God for healing.*

Later that afternoon Carolyn came into the room and suggested that Earl get himself something to eat at one of the restaurants near the hospital. He didn't want to leave me, but Carolyn assured him I would be all right and that she would introduce me to some of the other ladies on my floor.

I told Earl I would be okay while he was gone, so he kissed my forehead and hesitantly walked out the door.

"I appreciate your offer," I told Carolyn, "and I would like to meet some of the other ladies here. But I'm not quite ready to leave the room yet."

She looked at me with suspicion, so I quickly explained. "I'd like to visit with Flo for a while first."

I knew Flo was all alone and terribly ill. At that moment something inside of me began to change. Instead of wanting to run from Flo, my heart, mind and emotions shifted back to the caregiver that I always had been. In spite of my own poor health and weakness, maybe I could muster up enough energy and strength to care for this sweet, dear woman. I approached her bedside and asked if she would like me to read some scriptures. She smiled and nodded. I read to her several passages that I had found comforting, hoping God's words would somehow reach into her frail, pain-filled heart.

Her cloudy eyes filled with moisture as she looked up at me and breathed "Thank you" in a soft, weak voice. I spent the next thirty minutes talking with Flo, and discovered that she had never asked Christ into her life. It was becoming clear to me why I had been Divinely appointed to room 449B. I could tell Flo was getting tired, so I told her we would talk more about Christ at a later time, if she desired. She smiled and drifted off to sleep.

I left the room and headed down the hall to the visitation area, where several ladies had gathered. I entered the room apprehensively and the chatter stopped.

"Hi," I said with as much cheer as I could muster. "I'm Linda Harriss. I'm new on the unit and I thought I'd just come down and say hello to everyone."

For a moment, no one spoke. The silence threatened to suffocate me, but I stubbornly stood my ground.

Finally, a thin, pale, dark-haired woman sitting at the table said, "My name's Beth." She looked about thirty years old, although it was difficult to tell people's ages when their bodies were ravaged by this strange disease. "That's Jennie over there." Beth pointed to a pretty, middle-aged lady with beautiful silver hair and crystal-blue eyes. She sat alone in a corner chair, wiping tears from her eyes. "This is Debbie." Beth tilted her head toward a tall, beautiful young woman with long, dark brown hair and blue eyes.

Why, she can't be over twenty-one years old, I thought.

Debbie sat across the table from Beth, her chair tilted back on two legs, arms folded tightly across her chest. She glared at me and did not return my "hello."

"And that's Joan," Beth introduced. Joan stood near the television set, which had been vented to the outside to avoid filling the room with any toxic release. She was tall, probably 5'7", and looked to be a few years younger than me. Her reddish brown hair and green eyes were striking. Joan laughed at something on the TV, completely ignoring my presence.

"My husband, Earl, went out for a bite to eat," I said, slipping into an empty chair next to Beth. "So I thought I'd come down and meet each of you."

"Good for you," Joan commented with a sneer. "Must be nice to have a husband who hangs around when the going gets tough."

"You'll have to forgive her," Jennie whispered from her corner. "She's feeling very angry right now."

"Her husband just filed for divorce," Debbie explained. Her blue eyes flashed at Beth. "He couldn't handle this bizarre illness any better than the rest of our husbands," Joan added with a wry laugh. "They just can't take the responsibility of caring for us long term. When the doctor told my husband about all the changes that needed to be made in our lives and our home, he just flat-out refused to live like that."

I was in shock. I couldn't imagine what my life would be like if Earl abandoned me in this hour of my greatest need. "But surely you must have other family," I suggested.

"Sure," Joan said. "I have two kids, ages six and eight. They live with their dad in what used to be my home, in Chicago. That's an awful long way from Houston."

"How long have you been here?" I asked.

"In this hospital, almost three months," she said. "But I've had to stay here in Houston, to be near my doctor, for almost two years."

Jennie, I learned, was the veteran, having been in some form of isolation for three years. Debbie had suffered with Environmental Illness for just under a year; Joan for nine months. They sounded like prison terms to me.

"Where have you been living," I asked, "when you're not in this place?"

Beth shrugged. "I rent a room from another patient who was hospitalized here a couple of years ago."

"The hospital keeps a list of environmentally ill people who take in boarders," Joan informed me, her eyes never leaving the television screen.

"Don't you have any friends who are not afflicted with this condition?" I asked. These women's lives seemed far too focused on their disease.

"No one understands our illness," Debbie said, bringing the front legs of her chair down to the floor with a crashing sound that echoed in the bare room.

Jennie crept out of her corner and joined us at the table. "People are afraid. What happened to us is completely outside their realm of personal experience."

"You heard of that new AIDS virus?" asked Joan, glancing at me briefly during a commercial.

"Yes," I replied. "I'm a registered nurse."

"It has something to do with the immune system, right?" Beth asked.

"Yes," I answered, grateful for an opportunity to help these women in some small way.

"Well," Debbie said, "lots of people seem to think that's what we've got."

"That's ridiculous," I replied.

"Maybe," Beth said. "But folks are just as scared of us as if we had AIDS."

"Might as well be lepers," Joan said, reaching over to change the channel.

An awkward pause followed. Contrary to my normally chatty nature, I couldn't think of a single thing to say.

"Beth's going in for surgery next month," Jennie finally chipped in.

"Yeah," Beth freely admitted. "I have to have my colon removed." She shook her head. "Like being a Universal Reactor isn't bad enough, I'm dealing with cancer too!"

"Aren't they afraid you'll have an allergic reaction to the anesthesia?" I asked.

"Oh, the doctor tested me for several different meds. They're gonna use the one that showed the least amount of allergic sensitivity." Beth rolled her eyes at the ludicrous situation. "He said I'll still probably be really sick for several days after the surgery."

I had been wondering which was worse, cancer or Environmental Illness. Beth had the "winning answer"—both!

"Hey, Joan," Debbie suggested, "why don't you tell Linda how you got chemically exposed."

Joan turned off the TV set and joined the rest of us at the table. "My husband and I—we're separated now—purchased a new mobile home when we got married," she began. "After being in it for just a couple of months, I started to feel bad. Nausea, constant headaches, respiratory infections, depression—just to name a few. I developed asthma, too, which I'd never had before. The doctor said the building materials in my mobile home contained a lot of formaldehyde and other chemicals that overloaded my system."

"That sounds a lot like what happened to me," I said. I didn't really want to go into the details of my own exposure. As it turned out, I didn't have to. One by one each lady in the group eagerly shared her personal experience with Environmental Illness.

"I worked as a teacher for several years," Beth said." I developed chemical overload and several other allergies because of the schools' overuse of toxic cleaning supplies and pesticides." She explained that her room was in a portable building that had formaldehyde and mold in it, causing her system to crash because it couldn't handle the exposure. In fact, most schools have inadequate ventilation, leaving the air quality very poor. "I started having seizures in class one day. From that day on my symptoms of aches, pains, headaches, congestion, and seizures got worse."

Debbie had worked in a large manufacturing plant that exposed her to a lot of dangerous chemicals. "Several of my coworkers got cancer," she said.

"Dr. Morlen told me about that," I chimed in. "When people are exposed to chemicals for an extended period of time, their immune system is weakened, leaving them with a greater potential for developing various types of diseases and illnesses."

Jennie sat quietly in her seat, staring at the chair she'd vacated in the corner like she wanted to disappear into it.

"Come on, Jennie," Debbie prodded. "Tell Linda your story. We've all told her ours."

Jennie dabbed at her eyes with a white cotton handkerchief. "My husband and I remodeled our home. We replaced all the carpeting, peeled off the old wallpaper and put on a fresh coat of paint throughout the house. We added a new fireplace in the living room. Midway through the remodeling, I began experiencing chest pains, blurred vision, an ongoing low-grade fever, mental confusion, trembling, and heart palpitations. Every time I ate I became gravely ill."

I can certainly relate to that, I thought.

Jennie dabbed her eyes again, then added, "At first, I dismissed the symptoms, figuring my body was just responding to my stressful life and exhaustion. Then one evening, after being in the new living room for several hours, I collapsed on the floor. That's when we discovered that the gas burner in our new fireplace had a small leak. Dr. Morlen said the chemicals in the building supplies, combined with the gas leak, caused my immune system to collapse."

After Jennie completed her story, everyone stared at me. I wanted nothing more than to change the subject, to talk about something, anything, besides our chemical illness. But this weird disease seemed to be all these women had left in their lives. When family and friends had deserted you, and you lived in total seclusion for months or years on end, with virtually no contact with the outside world, there just didn't seem to be much else to talk about. These women hung on to their illness as if it helped them maintain some sort of personal identity. Or maybe they had accepted their illness and changes that had taken place in their lives. I couldn't. I had to keep fighting to get my life back.

"Where will you go when it's time to leave this place?" I asked, trying to direct the conversation to a subject outside these dull gray walls.

"I don't have any place to go," Jennie said flatly. "My husband divorced me—a year ago last Tuesday." Jennie scrambled back to her corner chair and curled up into it, sobbing quietly.

"I'm trying to get disability," Debbie said. "I gave that company I worked for everything I had. Now they're going to give me something. I've applied for Workman's Compensation. It'll be tough, though, because no one understands this crazy illness. Nobody believes my disability is work related. I get so tired of being misunderstood."

"Me and Joan are going to move to Alpine," Beth said. "There's a special community out there built just for us environmentally ill folks."

"They've converted a bunch of trailers to make them chemically free," Joan explained.

"It's in a nice rural area a few hundred miles southwest of here," Beth added.

"You make it sound like paradise," Debbie complained. "They're just tiny little camping trailers, with one room and a bath."

"There's a kitchen facility, too," Beth said defensively. "It's separated from the house trailers, to cut down on food odors."

"There's an outdoor cooking area, too," Joan added, "for those of us who are too sensitive to even enter the kitchen. Everyone uses electric grills for cooking."

Beth leaned her elbows on the table, obviously anticipating this luxury existence. "Each occupant gets their own refrigerator near the kitchen, and they've got special washers and dryers."

"The trailer rooms even have televisions." This feature was obviously quite important to Joan. "The sets are placed in the windows, like an air-conditioning unit, so the backs are actually outside. That keeps the fumes and electromagnetic radiation from getting indoors."

"What else could anyone want?" Beth asked, as if she had just described a mansion in Beverly Hills with servants and indoor swimming pools.

I couldn't hold my tongue any longer. "What else? How about a life?" I hated to burst their happy bubble, but I couldn't imagine living like that. "You have to be able to get out and go places and see other people once in a while. It's not natural to live like a hermit." After hearing their words, panic and fear took hold. *I cannot and will not accept what they are saying. I will not allow this to happen to me.*

"I know some folks with Environmental Illness," Jennie said quietly from her corner chair, "who haven't been able to leave their homes for ten years, except for doctor visits."

"I'd hate to become a prisoner in my own home," I said. "That would be like a death sentence."

The room grew quiet. Everyone seemed lost in their own thoughts, staring at the floor or the table or the walls. "I've put a gun to my head more times than I can remember," Debbie finally said, her voice pensive.

"I've wanted to end my life too," added Joan.

"We all have, at one time or another," Beth admitted. "The pain and the hopelessness get so intense. At the moment it seems the only way out of the physical and emotional pain."

"I'm glad you didn't go through with it," I said, shocked at what my ears were hearing. Then I noticed an old, worn Bible sitting on the end of the table in front of Beth. I wondered why I hadn't seen it earlier.

"We were having a Bible study when you walked in," Beth said. Hearing this, I realized that there was a belief that we did share. If we were to ever be free from this illness, it would come through what God would do in our lives. Studying His Word would sustain and guide us on this journey to recapture our lives or walk with us through the Valley of the Shadow of Death.

I told them I was a believer too, and that I would like to participate in their Bible studies. They assured me they would be happy for me to attend.

Debbie leaned back in her chair again. "We're all just hoping that somehow, someday, God will intervene in our lives."

"In the meantime," Jennie said, "we just wait . . . and pray . . . and wait some more."

I knew how they felt. It seemed like I would have to conquer the whole world in order to survive. I felt very small and weak in comparison to the world. *God, how big are you? Are you bigger than the world?* Immediately John 16:33 came to mind. "Here on earth you will have many trials and sorrows. But take heart, because I have overcome the world" (NLT).

Enter Earl

"Hey, Babe." Earl's voice was like heavenly music to my ears. I rushed into his arms, clinging to him even more tightly than before he'd left. Then I introduced my husband to my new friends. They all looked at him like he was an alien or an ax murderer. We went back to my room.

"Jennie's so quiet and sad," I said to Earl. "Debbie is extremely bitter. Joan laughs a lot, but there's deep-seated anger in her sarcastic remarks."

Earl listened without comment, squeezing my hand and looking attentively into my eyes. Just having him near me brought such strength and comfort in my life.

"Visiting hours are over," Carolyn came in and announced, all too soon. "Sorry. Hospital rules forbid anyone to stay overnight with the patients."

The thought of Earl leaving brought a sudden attack of panic. But as he cradled me in his arms I had a tiny glimpse of peace. I trusted this man with my life and knew he would die for me.

"I wish I didn't have to leave," he whispered.

"You need to go back to work tomorrow." My medical expenses were mounting. The allergy clinic had checked with our insurance company before I saw Dr. Morlen the first time. They had promised to submit the proper forms, but informed us that almost all claims were automatically rejected by the insurance companies. I felt awful for placing my family under such terrible financial stress. I was afraid we would have to spend the money we were saving for the children's education on medical expenses. This fight may not be worth it. What if things never get better and we wasted all of our savings on me? I felt so guilty for what I was doing to my family. They didn't deserve this.

As I watched Earl walk out those cold metal doors, Satan bombarded me with thoughts of him dying. If something happened to my husband, no one would be able to take care of me. I couldn't survive without him. I hated being so dependent on others for my very life. *Please, God, protect Earl and keep him safe.*

The night was long. My brain was so swollen I had trouble falling sleep. The pressure made my head feel like it would explode, and I sought relief through prayer. *Thank you, Jesus, for my family.* Would I ever be able to live a normal life with them again? Or would this meaningless existence forever be my world? *God, if I can't really live again and my family has to go through this, please just let me come and be with you. This isn't living; it's just existing.*

I felt totally alone.

God, are you there?

God, do you care?

CHAPTER FOUR

TROUBLE AND SORROW

Death had its hands around my throat; the terrors of the
grave overtook me. I saw only trouble and sorrow. Then I
called on the name of the Lord: "Please, Lord, save me!"
—Psalm 116:3–4

MY FIRST NIGHT WAS GRUELING. I woke up at 2:00 in the morning, and after several moments of grogginess realized I had slept pretty well in these strange surroundings. Being in this pure environment certainly did seem to help my condition. My biggest discomfort was a stabbing hunger, but eating was a never-ending frustration for me. Every time I ate, I became ill and depressed . . . so I'd rather be hungry.

I drifted off again and dreamed I was healed and back at work as a school nurse. I was walking down the hall in the elementary building with about ten students following me to my office to get their eyesight and hearing checked. Just a normal day at my normal job. I smiled at my precious students as they chattered happily amongst themselves.

A cheerful "Good morning, Linda" pulled me out of my dream and back into my living nightmare. "My name's Jo. I'm your new nurse."

The image of ten happy children was replaced by the sight of a tall, slim woman with freckles and brown hair wearing a bright white uniform. The jolt back to reality pierced my heart. Tears rolled down my cheeks and I couldn't speak.

"I need to get your vital signs." She slipped a thermometer under my tongue, then took my blood pressure and pulse. After she had recorded the results, she sat on the bed beside me. "Would you like me to pray with you?" she asked.

I nodded. *Thank you, Lord, for sending me a Christian nurse today.*

Jo prayed a beautiful, encouraging prayer, then squeezed my hand. "Linda," she said, "I really sense that the Lord is going to deliver you and that He has a special plan for your life."

Her words lit a tiny spark of hope in my heart, but my eyes saw little hope around me. Luke 1:37 came to my mind: "For nothing is impossible with God " (NLT). *Lord, I'm choosing to trust you. But sometimes I get so afraid.*

"None of your food-allergy testing can begin until you've completed your four-day fast," Jo reminded me. Dr. Morlen had originally wanted to make it eight days, but I was already so weak he didn't think I'd make it that long without food. "During your fast, we'll perform skin testing to determine how allergic you are to various substances other than food. The tests will take several days to complete, since Dr. Morlen has ordered you to be checked for just about every substance we test for."

That figures, I thought. I turned my head and winced as she stuck the needle into my vein.

"After learning how allergic you are to various things, we'll determine the optimal treatment dose for each substance."

I closed my arm against a fresh, dry cotton ball, and Jo led me down the hall toward the testing rooms. I followed her like a lost, frightened child.

"Your first allergy test will be for cotton," she said, referencing the magic fabric from which everything in this ward, from the nightgowns to the pillows and mattresses, was made.

I stopped in the middle of the hallway and stared at my white pajamas. "Do you mean I might even be allergic to these?" I asked. What was I supposed to do, walk around naked all the time? "And what about the cotton ball you used for my CBC?"

"For most people, cotton is less reactive than synthetic materials," Jo said. She looked at me with compassion. "I'm afraid there are some things that can't be avoided. You have to wear something." She opened one of the testing-room doors and led me inside. The far wall was lined with tables full of trays holding hundreds of small glass vials.

"These vials contain allergens," Jo explained. "They're actually various substances people can be allergic to."

"You're going to purposely inject me with things I'll probably get sick from?" *What kind of a house of torture was this place?*

"This is how we determine what your allergies are." She motioned for me to take a seat. "Based on our findings, we can prepare antigens for you that will help your body build up antibodies to combat your specific allergies."

Jo strolled toward the door. I felt like my only friend in the world was deserting me. "One of the testers will call you up to the appropriate table when she's ready for you." Jo smiled and left.

A Long Day of Testing

I stared at a long, rectangular table where other patients sat. Several were gathered at one end comparing stories of how they became chemically exposed. I took a chair at the opposite end of the table where I would be alone, because I couldn't bear to hear them repeat, over and over again, the stories of how they became ill. The only story I wanted to share about this illness was how God set me free from it. This place reeked of death and I wanted no part of it. I just wanted my life back.

"Harriss," a tired nurse behind one of the tray tables called.

I approached her like a condemned prisoner about to receive a lethal injection. She injected a small amount of the allergen under the skin on my right arm. Within seconds of the test my head and chest started to tighten. The pain became excruciating.

How can I be allergic to cotton? I wanted to crawl under the table and cry.

"What do we do now?" I asked through the fog of my pain.

"We have to wait and see if there's any reaction on your skin," she said, taking a seat beside me.

"How long do we wait?" I asked.

"After ten minutes we'll measure your reaction with this," she explained, showing me a device that looked like a ruler broken down into centimeters. "I'll record the measurement in your chart. That will help us find the right dose to treat you with."

She set a timer for ten minutes. "In the meantime, you need to tell me what symptoms you experience and the degree of severity. I'll record that too."

I felt miserable from head to toe pretty much all the time.

A nurse in the testing room injected me with allergens until 11:30, when the lab closed for lunch. Even though I was fasting, I was grateful for the break.

"We'll see you back here at 1:00, all right?" the nurse said with a smile.

"I can hardly wait," I responded.

From 1:00 to 4:30 I was tested for environmental irritants: trees, weeds, grasses, and such. After every test my throat tightened, I had shortness of breath, and I felt extremely lightheaded.

When the day's grueling tests were finally completed, I returned to my room, curled up on my bed, and tried to escape in sleep. But my body was in too much pain to rest. I sat up on my bed and opened the Word, but my mind had trouble focusing. I had to find a way to do something meaningful with my life. The one thing I've always enjoyed in the past was trying to help and comfort others. I got up and tried to share some Scriptures with Flo, but she didn't seem to respond.

Where are you, Father? Are you even real? Satan battled for control of my mind. *The enemy is always trying to steal your words away from me, Lord, tempting me to doubt your existence.* I turned to the Psalms and saw this verse: "I have hidden your word in my heart that I might not sin against you" (Psalm 119:11). I was grateful for the many years I'd had to study God's Word and learn about Him. *Thank you for a mother who made sure her children were always in churches where the gospel was proclaimed!*

As I lay in bed praying, I felt the Lord telling me to go to Beth's room and pray with her. Beth's kindness in welcoming me on my first day and introducing me to the other women in the Bible study had meant a great deal to me. I started down the hall. As I neared Beth's room, I heard sobbing and peeked through the doorway. There she was, sitting on the bed with a red nose, weepy eyes and several soiled tissues beside her. She looked frightened and alone. I asked her if she wanted me to pray with her.

"I'd like that," she said with a sniffle.

After a long, tearful time of prayer, Beth grabbed my hand and held it tight. She told me she'd been having a lot of abdominal pain, nausea, and vomiting. "There's blood in my stools too," she confessed in a whisper. It frightened her to think that the symptoms might indicate a serious progression of her colon cancer.

I encouraged Beth to tell her doctor about her symptoms when he came by on his rounds. She promised me she would. "I hope you don't mind," she added, "but I told another patient about you."

I wonder what she told her?

"Glenda's about your age and she's been sick for three years now. She's bedfast and has to be fed through feeding tubes because her body trembles so badly all the time."

Just like Flo.

"Besides," Beth added, "she's so depressed about her condition, she won't eat anymore."

"What did you say to her about me?" I asked, not sure I wanted to know.

"That you're a Christian and a strong woman of faith."

I couldn't decide whether I should feel flattered or scared. I sure didn't feel qualified to live up to such a reputation.

"Do you think you could go pray with her, like you did earlier today with me?" asked Beth.

Lord, do I have to? I remembered how frightened I was when I saw Flo for the first time. It was one thing to pray with someone like Beth, and I was doing the best I could with Flo, but what if Glenda was as ill as Flo? I really don't want to see another reminder of looming death. I wanted to surround myself with healthy, or at least healing, people—not dying ones! Besides, I'd been reading scripture to Flo for days and wasn't even sure she heard a word I said.

Some "strong woman of faith" I turned out to be. I made a concession and promised to pray for Glenda, and would certainly pray with her if I felt God leading me to do so . . . or if she called me to specifically ask for prayer. Thankfully, Beth seemed to understand my hesitation and didn't press the matter.

The evening following my first day of testing, Dr. Morlen came in with test results. "I'm not sure you'll be able to return to your home, Linda," he announced.

What? I was too stunned to speak, but just sat there in horror.

"Many of your chemical levels are extremely high. Your blood tests show your DDT level is off the charts. And you are especially sensitive to petroleum products."

I thought back to my childhood and how we played in the fog emitted from the mosquito spraying truck. The toxin in the spray was DDT. Little was known at that time about the harmful effects of chemicals on the human body. There certainly was no warning from officials to avoid contact with the toxic chemical. Dr. Morlen explained that chemicals can remain in our tissues for a lifetime and that, most likely, the DDT in my body was partially from the early years of my life. I began to understand the connection between the high disease rate and the use of chemicals in our world. I thought of my home in Brownwood that sat in the middle of fields containing a couple of oil and gas wells.

"The gas fumes from those wells will continue to destroy your immune system—what little of it that's left."

This was crazy. *God, you sent us to Brownwood and gave us our home. Why would you allow everything to be taken away from us now?*

"What am I supposed to do?" I asked in a daze. "Move to the desert and live in one of those special trailers like Joan and Beth?"

"That would be the best thing for you," he said. "It would allow minimal exposures to the chemicals that are prevalent in most modern environments."

I was in complete shock. I simply could not comprehend the magnitude of my situation. I certainly couldn't begin to fathom what my life would be like if I had to remain in isolation forever. That thought scared me more than anything.

"I won't leave my home and be separated from my family."

"The only possible alternative would be for your husband to provide a 'safe room' for you in your home. He would have to take everything out of the room. Everything." Dr. Morlen paused and looked me in the eye. "And there are no guarantees that it would work."

"There must be something we can do to fix all this."

"We'll continue the series of allergy shots we started when you first came to my office. But we'll make certain adjustments in them, once we have a better understanding of your immune system. We'll try to build up your tolerance as much as possible to as many things as we can."

"If I do all that, I'll get better, right?" I asked.

Dr. Morlen hesitated. "I must be honest with you, Linda. Most likely, you will always have a limited life."

A limited life? The phrase echoed through my addled brain. *A limited life? What was that supposed to mean?*

It was all so bizarre, I couldn't even begin to understand what was happening to me. I'm not sure I even wanted to. If it wasn't for the hope I had in Christ, I wouldn't have lasted one more day.

After Dr. Morlen left, my daughter, Christie, called. She had just gotten home from cheerleading practice and sounded so excited about it. This was her freshman year in high school. How I had looked forward to sharing these fun new experiences with her.

Thank you, Father, that Christie has something to be happy about today.

I spoke to Earl, too, and he tried to encourage me. When he started talking about all the things he knew I would be able to do again, I started crying. I felt completely overwhelmed. I knew he was trying to help me feel better, but his words only reminded me of all the things I would no longer be able to do. Had he forgotten what the doctor said? It's so much easier to believe when you aren't the person in the middle of a crisis.

Thank you, God, for a husband who loves me and still believes, even when I can't.

Second Day of Testing

The night was long, and I slept little. I woke up the next morning severely depressed. There was not another ounce of fight left in me. I was exhausted mentally, physically, and spiritually and didn't think I could live like this another second. But what were my alternatives?

No one understands me anymore. I don't even understand myself. How did my life change so quickly? Will I ever be happy again? Will I ever be me again? What happened to my life that was so full of fun and vitality? Will this disease turn me into such a strange person that no one will love me or want to be with me?

I came across Philippians 1:21: "For to me, to live is Christ and to die is gain." I'd been so incredibly spent and desolate, but now realized God was instructing me to share the scripture with Flo. I couldn't tell if she was coherent enough to understand what I read. But, I wanted her to know the life she could have with Christ living in her, and even if she died she would gain the magnificence of eternity.

Though at times depression swept over me like a consuming fire, leaving me feeling that death was the only way to end my pain, deep inside I didn't really want to die. I just wanted to be a part of life again. So I approached the day's testing with a renewed sense of determination.

It didn't last long.

The morning was frustrating and slow. After every injection I became so violently ill that they had to let my reactions subside for a long while before they could administer the next test.

The nurse shook her head and frowned each time she tested me. *I wonder if she realizes how my spirit is crushed each time she does that.*

"I want to do a chest X-ray on you today," Dr. Morlen informed me just before lunchtime.

"A chest X-ray?" I asked, thoroughly confused. "What for?"

"I want to check on those three large spots we found on your lungs when you were in my office the first time." With everything that was going on, I forgot about them. Would I be diagnosed with cancer, like Beth? How much of this could one human being be expected to handle all at once?

Please, Lord, don't let me have lung cancer, too!

I went through the motions in a fog of despair. During the lunch break I wandered back to my room and watched in silence as a nurse fed Flo her meal. I stared out the window and watched all the cars speeding up and down the highway. I wondered where they were all going.

Freedom itself had slipped away from me. *Will I always be staring out a window, never again part of the real world? I don't want to be a caged animal the rest of my life.* Envy threatened to consume me. I felt trapped by helplessness. God's Word was my only comfort and hope. "Be still before the Lord and wait patiently for him," I read in Psalm 37:7.

It would be so easy to just give up and die, Lord. But your Spirit deep inside me won't let me do that. I know you must have a plan for my life.

I endured more testing that afternoon. Dr. Morlen returned just before dinnertime with the results of my chest X-rays. He reported that the spots were completely gone. *Thank you, Lord!* I was grateful for this blessing, but still could not understand why God would make the spots on my lungs disappear while leaving me with this strange, complex illness.

That night, Dr. Morlen told me he had decided to shorten my fast. "Your immune system is weaker than I originally thought," he said. "You are severely hypersensitive to everything we've tested you for thus far. So I've decided to go ahead and start your food-allergy tests first thing tomorrow."

I went to sleep that night with one thought on my mind: I could finally eat again! I wondered if the food would make me sick, but still looked forward to breakfast. Day three had arrived and I was hungry. But, when the tray arrived the next morning, I was acutely disappointed. There sat two large bowls of organic peas. Nothing else. Just two bowls full of tiny green pellets. I hadn't expected steak and eggs, but I was sure hoping for something a bit more appetizing to "break my fast."

"Why peas?" I asked the nurse who had brought in my tray.

"We haven't tested you yet for food allergies," she said as she fed Flo her oatmeal. "We have to feed you something."

I hope that organic peas aren't the only thing I can tolerate! I thought.

The nurse scooped a spoonful into Flo's mouth. "There's really no way to predict how reactive you'll be until you start your allergy tests."

I was too famished to argue, so I gobbled down every last pea. Within minutes, my body started shaking, my head began pounding, and I had trouble breathing. Organic peas! Will there be anything my body won't react to?

Nurse Jo came in after breakfast and took me back to the testing room.

"Our first priority today," she explained, "is to test for foods that people normally react to least. That way, you can start eating and trying to put some weight back on as soon as possible."

Sounded good to me. I was tired of looking emaciated. Besides, there had to be more to life than organic peas.

I was tested for various food allergies all morning long. Beef caused my chest to tighten till I couldn't breathe. Corn put my brain into a mental fog. Milk made me incredibly sleepy. Cane sugar put me into a severe depression and made my hands and body tremble violently. Chicken was the only food that didn't cause a major reaction.

I devoured my all-too-small portion of baked chicken for lunch. It was tasteless and dry, and I had to wash it down with big gulps of spring water. Knowing that I could eat without fear of allergic reaction made the sparse meal seem like a feast! But shortly after I finished eating, my usual symptoms began to return. Thankfully, the reaction was mild compared to other times. I thanked the Lord that at least there was something I wasn't severely allergic to!

After lunch, my food-allergy testing continued. My file grew quickly as the technician recorded all my reactions. I was sure she would have writer's cramp by the end of the day.

One other food was found to be "safe" for me: fish. That evening, I had broiled fish for dinner. For such a bland food, it tasted wonderful to me. And I had no allergic reaction to it! None! Fish suddenly became the basis of my diet. I recalled Grandmother's dream about the illuminated fish and the Lord telling her not to touch it because it was part of my healing. I smiled and told myself, "God, really does have a plan for my life. And He wanted to show me that He has every detail of my life under control."

After dinner Dr. Morlen returned with more test results. And more bad news.

"Linda," he told me, "you are even more allergic now than when I first tested you in my office two months ago. Your immune system continues to go down."

God, you're going to have to pull off a big one to get my life together. But you created my immune system, so you can repair it. You can, can't you?

"It's a good thing you came into the hospital when you did so you could get more thorough allergy testing. Now that we know about your immune system and reactions, your allergy shots will be customized to benefit you more."

After Dr. Morlen left, I sat on my bed in a state of emotional numbness. *Lord, this disease is so cruel. But I'm reminded of how cruel your death was. Thank you for what the cross means in my life. Whether I live or die, I know my sufferings will be worth it all when I enter into your presence.*

I had always cared about others, but sometimes I couldn't understand what they were going through. Amazing how significant pain can be when it becomes personalized. I didn't like it one bit!

Something deep in my spirit was telling me to relinquish self-sufficiency and control, and I knew I had to trust Him no matter where life's pathways took me. But still . . . trusting was hard at this time in my life. But I would work hard to try.

I began reading Scripture to Flo, but was interrupted by a phone call. It was Glenda, the patient Beth had talked to about me.

"Could you come see me?" she asked, her voice hoarse and frail. "Please?"

I remembered my promise to Beth that I would pray with Glenda if she asked me to.

Opportunities To Minister

My head still throbbing from the day's testing, I shuffled to Glenda's room. Along the way I tried to mentally and emotionally prepare myself to meet another patient whose Environmental Illness was as severe as Flo's. *Lord, I would rather die than become an invalid like Glenda or Flo. I didn't want my family to have to take care of my every need.*

I braced myself and entered Glenda's room.

The woman was thin and frail, much like Flo. She looked like a skeleton—pale and lifeless and literally wasting away in her dark and gloomy room. I asked if I could turn the lights on, but she groaned a negative response. As I approached her bed, I realized she was sobbing. Then as soon as I introduced myself, she began speaking.

"Joey called me tonight," she whispered through tears. "He's my nine-year-old son," she explained. "He asked me if there really is a God. Before I could answer, he told me there couldn't be a God because He hasn't answered his prayers."

I asked her if Joey had ever given his heart to Jesus.

"Yes," she replied.

"I can sure understand why he might feel discouraged," I said. "Satan brought those same thoughts to my mind just a couple of days ago. And I've been a believer for twenty-four years. How much easier it must be for a child to doubt God's existence and His love."

Glenda seemed to relax a bit, and I thought I saw the hint of a smile.

"Joey is just afraid and confused right now," I assured her. "But in his heart he knows there's a God because the Lord is in his heart."

I knew my own children must be having a lot of doubts, just like Glenda's son. I prayed I would never say or do anything that would turn them away from God. *We all need you so badly, Lord. Reassure Joey, Greg and Christie that you are there. Please assure me too.*

We prayed together for our children and I shared Mark 9:24: "Lord, I believe; help thou mine unbelief" (KJV). Glenda hugged me and thanked me for praying with her. Her eyes and her smile shone brightly. As I left her room, I realized that even when I didn't want to and had nothing left to give, I could still give others hope through prayer and God's Word.

Visitors!

It was now the evening of the third day of testing. I could hardly sleep that night, anticipating the weekend. I would have to face more tests the next morning (Saturday), but would get a reprieve in the afternoon and on Sunday receive visitors. The days had gone by so slowly and it felt like a life-time since I'd seen my family or friends.

The night was torturous and long. I felt and watched every second go by. Bright and early Saturday morning the charge nurse came in to check on me. To my utter humiliation, I recognized her as a woman I had gone through nursing school with. Dorothy seemed as shocked to see me lying in that bed as I was to see her walk through the door of my room. We both just stared at each other. I wanted to run and hide. It was embarrassing that I was no longer the person she had known in nursing school. My personality had changed from happy and outgoing to depressed and withdrawn. My once healthy appearance was now emaciated and fragile.

"Linda?" she asked hesitantly. "Linda Harriss?"

Having Dorothy see me in such a weak and helpless state was demoralizing.

"Didn't you go to nursing school at Tarleton State University?" she asked.

No! I wanted to shout. I was not the same person Dorothy had gone to nursing school with—the competent woman who was elected both class president and class representative at the same time. I had been the student liaison with the nursing school faculty. I had studied hard, made good grades, and organized class events, parties, and study groups.

Fighting back tears, I replied in a quivering voice, "Yes, I'm that Linda Harriss."

After a moment's hesitation, she said, "I'm so sorry." With a look of shock and disbelief, she took my vital signs and left the room. But later she came back to my room to apologize for her quick departure.

"I just didn't know what to say. I was so shocked to see you in this condition," she explained.

I reassured her and accepted her apology, because I certainly didn't understand this illness either. We hugged and she left the room, still appearing to be in shock.

I buried my head under the covers until it was time for my testing to begin.

My first allergy test of the morning caused a severe and immediate reaction. My brain swelled so much it felt like my skull would crack open. Dr. Morlen explained to me that I had cerebral allergies. My brain was locked into *fight or flight* mode and saw everything that I came in contact with as an enemy. Due to this reaction that took place in my brain, my whole body was affected—from heart palpitations, severe headaches, changes in mood, depression and insomnia, to shortness of breath and others. *Why couldn't I have normal reactions like a runny nose or rashes?*

As I sat in that testing room, waiting and praying for the pain to subside, I felt completely alone. I no longer had anything in common with anyone. My world was so different from everyone else's. I just wished they would all forget me and let me die. Then I wouldn't be a burden to anyone.

Two hours later, the pain finally began to decrease.

"We won't do any more testing today," the nurse decided, much to my relief. "Your family's coming today, and you don't want to feel so bad that you can't enjoy their visit."

Sure enough, my sister Delores called to tell me that she and Sonny were coming to see me later in the afternoon. Earl and the kids and my mom were due to arrive at noon, which meant I had an entire hour to wait.

I sat on my bed and stared at the clock, then walked down the hall and stood as close to the entry doors as I could. Watching every single one of those sixty minutes pass by, I peered through the glass windows on the door as if I could will my family to arrive early. When I saw them step out of the elevator, my heart started racing. I brushed away the tears that threatened to overtake me because I didn't want to upset Greg and Christie. When they entered the doors into the reception area, a nurse went up to them right away to make sure they weren't wearing anything that had a scent. They knew the hospital rules and were quickly given approval to enter.

The moment we saw each other, we all shared hugs and words of "I love you" and "I've missed you." I wanted to say, "I'm so sorry for the pain I've created in your life," but I bit back the words. I didn't want to draw attention to the sadness we were already feeling. So I led my family back to my room, aware of the discomfort and fear in Christie's and Greg's eyes as they looked around the room. When other severely ill and fragile looking patients passed, my children's nervousness grew worse.

Working hard to put on brave faces, Christie and Greg shared with me what was going on in their lives. They spoke about all the exciting things they were doing. They were swimming a lot and spending the night with friends. Greg enjoyed roller skating and Christie was busy working out to get ready for volleyball season.

"We're playing in Breckenridge on Monday for our first preseason game," Christie announced. "We're leaving real early in the morning on the school bus."

My heart choked with excruciating pain as I realized that I was no longer part of their everyday world. With this realization, Satan managed to worm in a debilitating thought, and I bought into the gut wrenching lie that I needed them but they didn't need me. Their lives were going on while I sat in this lifeless hospital and shriveled away. I wouldn't for a second want their fun and excitement to be over just because mine was, but it hurt to think that I was no longer a vital, necessary part of their daily lives.

God, I can't take this alone. Please do something. I hate this isolation from life and my family.

When the kids and Mom went down to the hospital cafeteria to grab some lunch, I told Earl what Dr. Morlen had said. "I probably won't be able to live in our house ever again," I sobbed.

"If we have to," he said, "we'll move. We're going to do whatever it takes to get you well, Babe. If I need to sell everything we have, I'll do it."

Thank you, Father, for blessing me with Earl's presence in my life. His love and commitment to me is incredible. Such a reflection of your love for me. I don't know why he loves me, but I am so glad he does! Still, I knew I couldn't ask my family to leave our home.

"Christie and Greg have great friends, they're enjoying their school, and they're really involved in our church. I can't ask them to give all that up for me," I said, hating that I was taking so much from everyone, especially when I had nothing to give in return. I felt empty inside. Absolutely worthless to anyone.

Earl said we'd talk about it later. He kissed me, then went downstairs to have lunch with the kids and Mom. The moment he left my room, my heart sank to the pits of darkness and despair. It felt like my life was at a standstill. Every moment seemed filled with nothing but pain, fear, and frustration.

This is all so cruel. Have I done something terrible to deserve this?

I thought about all the children I had worked with as a school nurse. Many were abused, some by their own mothers and fathers. It angered me to know that while child abusers walked about freely, I was imprisoned by this insanely restrictive illness.

It all seemed so unfair.

Delores and Sonny

On Saturday my sister Delores and her husband Sonny arrived while Earl and the kids were downstairs. I was elated to see them. Delores' eyes filled with tears the second she saw me. She grabbed my hand and said, "Is there anything I can do? Anything at all? I've been so worried about you." I knew she desperately wanted to help and was very sad and frustrated at my plight. It was frustrating for me too. I asked her to continue to pray, and she assured me she would. Sonny then prayed, asking the Lord to heal me. "I'm sorry you are going through this. It must be so hard on Earl and the kids too. We'll just keep praying and believing." he said, then gave me a hug.

When the rest of my family returned from their meal, they were thrilled to see Delores and Sonny. Since my allergy testing had been cut short and my symptoms had somewhat subsided and were not as severe, I was able to enjoy the visit. We all spent the rest of the day together chatting.

But through all the light conversation, my spirit felt crushed. My family was making incredible concessions for me, and still it wasn't enough! How could I ask everyone I knew to change their lives in such dramatic ways, just so they could spend a few minutes visiting with me? It seemed nearly everything in creation attacked my oversensitive immune system! I was overwhelmed by the feeling that the entire world had turned against me.

I don't know if I can handle all this, God. I can't control the whole world! Can you?

CHAPTER FIVE

AND ALL OF JOB'S FRIENDS SHOWED UP

I have become a laughingstock to my friends, though I called
on God and he answered.
—Job 12:4

THE TESTING LABS WERE CLOSED ON SUNDAYS. Never before had the "day of rest" concept held so much meaning! Although the hospital didn't offer worship services, I met briefly, first thing in the morning, with Beth and several other women in our unit for Bible study and prayer. It was a nice, quiet time and I appreciated these ladies a great deal. Still, I longed to be at my own church worshipping with my family and friends.

When I returned to my room, I asked Flo if she would like me to share with her the essence of the Bible study. She slowly nodded her head. Since she could not leave the room to join our study, she seemed to appreciate the opportunity to participate in this more individual, intimate way. We discussed Philippians 4:11, "For I have learned to be content whatever the circumstances." This was a difficult lesson for me; I knew it had to be doubly so for Flo in her bedridden and advanced state of the disease that plagued us both.

The doctor who was on call for the weekend came by. He introduced himself as Dr. Peterson. For some reason, I immediately started to cry. I felt so depressed. He tried to console me, but I couldn't stop weeping.

"I feel so hopeless," I tried to explain. "All of my allergy tests have come back positive. I seem to be allergic to the whole world."

He patted my hand and listened attentively. "Linda," he said, when I finished complaining, "it doesn't matter what the medical reports say. Ultimately, the Lord has the final word."

I couldn't believe what I was hearing. I never would have expected such Spirit-filled encouragement from an attending physician.

Lord, thank you for Christian doctors!

A Burden of Guilt

My life had always revolved around my children. Now I couldn't even be with them outside of this hospital room. Since it was Sunday morning, sadness washed over me because the weekend was coming to an end. Earl, Mom, Greg, and Christie would be going home in the afternoon. Monday would bring about their normal routines of work, school, and athletic activities.

Is this my reward for being a devoted mother? My love for them was unfathomable. I used to wonder how God could love them more. I saw being my children's mother as a blessing, and a responsibility to help guide, shape, and mold their lives. I always wanted to protect them from being hurt and keep them free of pain. Now I was struggling to care for myself. I clung to the belief that someday this terror would be over and I would be part of their world again. Holding on to my faith was my only hope. Some days were harder than others to keep on believing. I had to constantly remind myself that my emotions, which changed like the wind, could not overrule Truth. It isn't fair how something you have no control over can change almost everything about you in a matter of minutes.

When lunch arrived I was offered my choice of chicken or fish. I turned down both. I felt so bad already and didn't want to take a chance of food making me worse. My family went downstairs to the hospital cafeteria to grab a bite to eat, and then to the mall to purchase a few items for the children.

My older brother, Hughie, came to see me shortly after they left. He brought along my Uncle Wesley and Aunt Trudie. That should have really lifted my spirits, but my body reacted to something they were wearing. I went into a sudden and severe depression. Again, I felt terrible for inconveniencing everyone. Why did I have to be such a pain? I was grateful for their sacrifice, traveling from Pearland on a Sunday afternoon to visit me in the hospital. And I knew they had done their best to follow all the hospital's rules before visiting me. Yet, in spite of all their precautions, something had been missed or not understood, and here I was, reacting again! Depression shrouded me, preventing my mind from forming any kind of rational reasoning, and making a pleasant visit with my family difficult.

I felt strange—and embarrassed. I wondered what everyone was thinking about me. I hated seeing the look of pity in their eyes and didn't want anyone to know how badly I felt. I wanted to be well and healthy like everyone else.

This must be what people who are born with disabilities feel like when they are around those who are not disabled. I could understand their pain now in a way I never did before. I felt like death and laid on my bed like an invalid, feeling totally helpless and dependent on others. I hated that more than anything. My brother, Paul, called to encourage me. I could hear the sadness in his voice. He always had a heart full of love and compassion. Hughie, Wesley, and Trudie left after a couple of hours. I know it upset them to see me so lifeless. I felt so responsible for everyone's emotions. And I didn't like what I felt.

A few minutes later, my mom's voice filtered through the fog in my brain.

"Linda, Honey," she whispered, "Dad's here."

I looked up at my father's face and could see in his eyes that his heart was broken by what had happened to his little girl. But I knew he couldn't admit it or talk about it. He had never been able to express his feelings in words. I never doubted that he loved me, but spoken terms of endearment

—like "I love you"—were something he just could never bring himself to say.

So Dad sat quietly by my bed, holding my hand. He said very little, but his eyes spoke volumes of love. After a few minutes, those eyes started to mist up. Silently, he released my hand, got up quickly, and went out into the hall. As he stood alone outside my room, I saw his shoulders quiver and knew he was fighting tears.

Do-Gooders?

While they were gone, a woman arrived whom I vaguely recognized from an out of town church that I'd visited a couple of times. She was accompanied by another woman and two men. They introduced themselves as the Visitation Committee: Mary, Catherine, Wayne, and John. Their words were sympathetic and caring.

The purpose for their visit revealed itself quickly.

"We want to explain to you how you can receive healing," said Mary, a soft-spoken, petite redhead.

"It's quite simple, really," added John, a six-foot-tall man with black hair and brown eyes. "The Bible says that if you confess all of the hidden sin in your life, you can be healed."

I knew I hadn't lived a flawless life, but I had always tried to deal with my sins as soon as they occurred. "I've already confessed and re-confessed all the sins I can think of," I tried to explain.

"Then you must not have enough faith in God's ability to heal you," Wayne determined, settling his stout frame into a nearby chair.

"I don't think that's it, either," I argued. I knew God could heal me. I didn't understand why He hadn't yet, but it certainly wasn't because I didn't believe He could.

"It has to be one or the other," insisted Catherine. Her blue eyes bored into mine as if she were trying to make a judgment call on the spot. "All sickness and disease come about either from a lack of faith or from sin in a person's life."

That seemed awfully simplistic to me. If it were true, then God was being terribly cruel. I didn't like thinking of Him in those terms.

"You must have unshakable faith," Mary asserted with a curt nod.

Easy for her to say, I thought. Mary was probably in good health. I wondered how much faith she would have if she were fighting my battle.

"Just confess all the healing scriptures," John said. He handed me a pamphlet with a list of Bible verses. "Then claim that you are already healed and go about your life as if you were well."

How my mind wanted to do that! But my body wouldn't allow me to. I'd already tried "confessing all the healing scriptures" and going about my life as if nothing were wrong. I had lived that way for weeks before finally agreeing to be admitted to this hospital. I knew from experience that there had to be a lot more to it than that. What, I still wasn't sure. But these people didn't seem to have the answer.

Lord, why do I have to listen to all this? How can your children be so cruel?

"Look," I said, trying to remain cordial, "I'm feeling really depressed today, and these things you're saying aren't helping."

"Depression comes from Satan, you know," Wayne declared. "Never from our loving Lord. Only good things come from God."

"I know there are times when the enemy attacks us and we can feel sad and depressed," I cried. "And sometimes we're depressed because of traumatic things that happen in our lives. But my depression began when I was accidentally exposed to toxic chemicals. I know that is so hard to believe, but I'm not lying. My doctor said the chemistry and function of my brain changed when I got that toxic exposure. That's why I became depressed. My life was great before this happened."

"Linda, I've never heard of depression being caused by chemicals," Wayne replied. "That's just hard to believe. The enemy is just blinding you so you don't see the truth."

I was overwhelmed with feelings of failure. Apparently I wasn't good enough to receive a healing from God. I felt completely worthless before my loving heavenly Father. Was my whole Christian life just a lie? Had I fooled myself into thinking God loved me unconditionally and had accepted me just as I was?

As politely as I could, I said, "You just don't understand."

"We're just trying to help," Catherine said.

There was only one way I could think of that they could help. But none of them were volunteering to take my place.

"The blessed Lord will not put any more on you than He knows you can handle," Mary assured me.

I wondered if any of them would survive if they had to live my life for even one day. "Then why is He allowing me to be in so much pain?" I asked, wondering what delightfully pat platitude they would offer me.

"I do have faith, and I've already confessed every sin I have ever committed a zillion times," I repeated, my frustration growing apparent. "Besides, I thought the first time we ask forgiveness for our sins, God forgives us."

"Well, that is true . . ." Catherine conceded, a slight frown marring her fair complexion.

"Then I don't understand —"

"If you're going to be healed, it is really up to you," Mary interrupted, her chin lifting slightly. "Your healing is there. You just have to receive it." With that pronouncement, she prayed for me, and they exited my room. I knew their hearts and intentions were pure, but I wondered if they, literally or figuratively, shook the dust off their feet as they left, like Jesus instructed His disciples to do whenever someone "does not receive you, nor heed your words" Mathew 10:14 (NAS).

I wanted to cry. I felt so humiliated. Like a failure. At this point I realized that I had to decide to continue walking in faith or walk away from God forever. I felt tormented.

Satan attacked my mind immediately. What if they were right? Was God failing me? Was His Word true? Was He really there? Did He care about me at all? I felt completely rejected by God and His people. Even if He did exist, He couldn't possibly care what happened to me. If He loved me, He would have prevented this horrible nightmare, or at least would have healed me from it by now. Swallowed up by an intense sense of depression, frustration, and condemnation, once again I realized that I could have walked away from the Lord that instant and never returned to Him.

But in that moment, God reminded me of 1 Corinthians 2:4–5: "Not with wise and persuasive words, but with a demonstration of the Spirit's power, so that your faith might not rest on human wisdom, but on God's power." That passage helped calm down my intense despair a little and I clung to it with all I had. Again, I made the hard choice to believe what I had known to be true. *Lord, you are the Great Jehovah Rapha—my healer. You and you alone are my deliverer. Only you are God. Let me rest in your sweet peace and presence.*

Earl and the children returned after lunch. I knew my time with them was running short and I didn't want to upset them, so I didn't mention my visit from the "committee." We talked all afternoon until they left for dinner. As I lay quietly by myself, I began to reflect back over my visit from my well-meaning guests who made me question myself and God. Why was it so difficult for people to understand my pain, especially my depression, was caused by toxic chemicals, not sin in my life? I had to confess, though, that I'd often been guilty of thinking similar thoughts about others at various times. So many things in life are beyond our ability to comprehend. This disease certainly fit into that description.

Despair, frustration, and anger overtook me. How could anyone minimize my illness just because they had never experienced it? Everything within me wanted to unleash my anger on them, but I didn't have the energy and I knew it would be to no avail. Their minds were made up, and they would not see things differently. As I continued lying in my bed once again replaying the negative words spoken to me, I was reminded of the power of words. A person can be encouraged or destroyed by our words. We can speak life or death over someone else's life. *Lord, may I only speak words of life and love to those in my life, for as you say, "Death and life are in the power of the tongue"* (Proverbs 18:21, NKJV).

When Earl, Mom, and the kids returned from their dinner, I tried to act like everything was okay. But I was in too much pain. All too soon, it was time for them to leave, and I had to stay behind. My heart ached because they were leaving, and I was still feeling hurt by my last visitors. I approached this hurt and sadness, that they were leaving, as I had dealt with previous disappointments. I needed time to process my emotions before I could talk to my family. Besides, they were dealing with a lot of heavy emotions and they certainly didn't need to carry mine. I couldn't inflict more agony in their lives.

Christie hugged me and whispered, "I love you, Mom." Her words brought me a surge of joy. I couldn't hold back the tears. When she saw me cry, she fell into my arms and wept pitifully with me. Then she prayed, asking the Lord to heal me and allow me to return home soon. Greg and Earl tried to be strong. But I knew their hidden anguish.

Lord, please heal their hearts and take away their pain. I lift them up to you. Protect them, Father.

The moment they walked out those cold steel doors, I was once again overcome with guilt for the pain I had inflicted on the people I loved most. I sank into a severe depression and longed to be with my family for more than just a few hours a week.

If that's not possible, Lord, I just want to leave this world and be with you.

How quickly depression robbed me of my hope again!

More Testing

Monday morning brought the excruciating realization that I would not see my family again for another five days. I shuffled to the testing room like a robot on automatic pilot.

"Today," Nurse Jo said in a much-too-chipper voice, "we will began testing you for inhalants." She prepared the needle, and I placed my arm in the appropriate position. "Inhalants," she explained, "are airborne allergens. The most common are dust and mites. The testing will take three days. There are many inhalants that can be tested here, and Dr. Morlen requested that you be checked for all of them."

Of course he did.

"We'll be testing you for pollens, animal dander's, terpenes—"

"What in the world is a terpene?" I asked.

"Terpenes are hydrocarbons found in essential oils, resins, and balsams. They're especially prevalent in solvents, but they're also found in perfumes and other scented items like shampoo, soap, and deodorant."

Great. Not only am I supposed to walk around naked for the rest of my life, I have to be dirty and smelly, as well.

"Some people are extremely sensitive to odors from hydrocarbons, especially those found in oil, gas, and coal. They may react to tiny leaks of natural gas from the range, refrigerator, dryer, or water heater."

"We converted all our gas appliances to electric," I said, grateful that God had miraculously shown us how harmful gas was for me.

"Oh, leaking refrigerant gas from electric refrigerators can be an allergen, too," Jo said. "So can oil odors from the garage or furnace, from appliances with lubricated electric motors or fans, or from oil-soaked filters in air conditioners. Fumes from warm-air heating systems can also cause symptoms. Even steam heating can affect people who are susceptible to the odor of chlorine in water."

No wonder I react to everything!

I was tested from 9:00 in the morning until 11:30, then again from 1:00 until 4:00. Just like with the food-allergy tests, I reacted strongly to every inhalant I was tested for. I refused to eat lunch or dinner because I didn't want to add any more irritants to my system.

Dr. Morlen came in at the end of the day with even more bad news. "Your autoimmune test came back positive," he said.

"What does that mean?"

"I'm not sure right now. We'll have to retest you at a later time. Either you have lupus or your immune system is so bad that it has given us a false reading."

I should have been frightened by the possibility of having this condition. Perhaps I had had too much frightening news in a short period of time, but Dr. Morlen's pronouncement did not strike a single chord of fear in my heart. I reminded myself God has the final authority over life and death. I recalled 2 Corinthians 5:7: "For we live by faith, not by sight."

At the moment I could think clearly because my depression was not severe.

Spiritual Warfare

I awoke the next morning engaged in a terrible battle with my emotions. I just wanted to give up. And yet, it frightened me to even acknowledge that I felt that way. Satan again bombarded my mind. *"God doesn't really love you,"* he whispered. *"If He did, He would have already healed you!"*

I didn't want to believe such a horrible thought, but emotionally, I had nothing left to fight it. *"Why don't you just turn to me?"* Satan continued to whisper. *"I'll provide healing for you."* A verse came to my mind from somewhere, and I grabbed it like I was drowning. "Lord," I prayed in shock and desperation, "Hearing myself think this stuff terrifies me. I had no idea I could go there. Help me stay strong in you."

I laid claim to 2 Corinthians 10:5: "We demolish arguments and every pretension that sets itself up against the knowledge of God, and we take captive every thought to make it obedient to Christ."

Lord, I prayed, *as badly as I want healing, I realize that nothing is more important to me than my relationship with you. Please help me to remain committed to you no matter how tough the battle gets.*

Time for more tests. When I walked into the testing room, I knew I would probably have major reactions. But as long as I could sit up, I was determined to complete the testing as quickly as possible. I couldn't wait to get out of that hospital and back home with my family.

Greg called after dinner to tell me how much he loved and missed me. Once again, guilt overtook me. I had had horrible reactions to the testing. My emotions were shaky. As always, I hated that I caused my son pain.

"Please, Greg," I begged my son, tears making speech almost impossible. "Just try to forget you ever had a mom named Linda, okay?"

"What are you talking about?"

"If you forget about me, then you won't have to hurt so badly." I knew it would devastate me if my family forgot about me. But I would rather endure any amount of pain than inflict the smallest amount on my children and my husband.

"Mom," Greg said, "I could never do that. I love you too much to forget you."

"I love you with my whole heart. I'm so sorry that you are sad because of me."

I woke up the next morning terribly depressed and in extreme physical pain. I suffered through my final day of inhalants testing, then was told I would begin the series of tests for chemicals and molds first thing the following day.

"Those usually cause far more severe reactions than the inhalants," Jo forewarned me.

I wouldn't want my worst enemy to suffer like this. *When will the hurting end?*

That afternoon I got a call from a woman who introduced herself as Jill.

"A friend of mine told me about your illness," she said, her cheerful voice only making my depression worse. "She thought I would remember you from seeing you around the school, because you were always really involved in your children's sports and activities. My kids go to the same school as yours," she explained.

I didn't recall seeing Jill at any of the school functions, but I did remember working with her at the Brownwood Hospital a couple of times. I wondered why someone who wasn't even sure how she knew me was bothering to call. She didn't ask how I was doing, but seemed more interested in talking, so I let her.

"Anyway, when my friend told me your name was Linda Harriss, that rang a bell. I started piecing together the information and finally realized that I knew you from the Brownwood Hospital. I only saw you a couple of times there, but I remember you were so vibrant and full of life. I was shocked to hear you were sick. Then, when my friend told me you were actually fighting for your very life, well, I just had to call and tell you how sorry I am."

Great. Pity from someone who barely even remembers me.

Then she asked, "Didn't you used to be a nurse?"

Oh, how those words pierced my heart and soul! *Used to be.* I was just a "used to be."

I don't even know who I am anymore!

I squeezed a small "yes" out of my constricted throat, and Jill continued chattering. But those three words rang in my ears, drowning out her voice. *Used to be.* I could think of nothing except all the things I used to be that I would never be again.

Jill finally ran out of things to say and said good-bye. I sat on my bed and stared out the window. I wanted nothing more than to leave that sterile room and run outside in the sunshine smelling flowers and feeling the gentle breeze on my face. I asked God to forgive me for not being as sensitive as I should have been to those around me who were afflicted and unloved. Who am I to feel that perhaps others deserve pain, but not me?

I opened my well-worn Bible and read Isaiah 40:31: "Yet those who wait for the Lord will gain new strength; they will mount up with wings like eagles, they will run and not get tired, they will walk and not become weary" (NAS).

I reflected back on how my heart had been broken by harsh and judgmental words spoken to me by individuals who didn't understand my illness. The shame and guilt resulting from the verbal attacks shattered the core of who I was. I felt I had to not only fight my disease to live, but I had to fight to maintain my self-worth as well.

"Lord, help me to be mindful of my words spoken to others. May they be a reflection of your love."

The night was long. I didn't sleep for a moment, dreading the next series of tests.

Please, Lord, grant me mercy and grace to cope. I can't do this without your help.

CHAPTER SIX

DISEASED FROM LACK OF KNOWLEDGE

*Worship the Lord your God, and his blessing will be on your
food and water. I will take away sickness from among you . . .
I will give you a full life span.*
—Exodus 23:25–26

9:00 A.M. FINALLY ARRIVED, and I marched myself into the testing room, overwhelmed with a deep sense of sadness.

"Are you ready to start the new tests?" Jo greeted me.

Do I have a choice? I thought, as I fought tears.

"For the next three days," she continued, obviously taking my silence as acceptance, "we'll be testing you for various chemicals, hormones, and molds. Did you know there are twenty-six different kinds of mold?"

Who knew? And not sure I care?

"Chemical allergens are found in our homes, air, water, food and drink, drugs, cosmetics, and textiles," Jo told me. "They're also in the pesticides used to control insects in our homes and public places. They're hard to pinpoint because they're taken for granted and they permeate all aspects of society."

I didn't understand how such strange things could be happening to me. Just a short time ago I was perfectly healthy. How quickly and completely my life had changed. Nothing made sense anymore. I felt like a little child who had lost her way.

Chemical Sensitivity 101

According to Jo, allergens are found most commonly in carpeting and pads, upholstery, drapery, clothing, and bedding. But odors from synthetic materials, including soft plastics and vinyl, rubber, polyester, rayon, and nylon, can cause symptoms and illness, as can the chemicals found in solvents, dyes, and household cleaners including polishes, waxes, detergents, fabric softeners, and cleansers.

Since my symptoms were usually worse at night, it meant that I may be reacting to foam pillows and mattresses. Unfortunately, my symptoms were bad all the time, day and night.

Jo continued to share the complexity of my ailment. "People who suffer with chronic sensitivities may start out with mild, vague symptoms that together are severe enough to prompt them to see a doctor. They might feel fatigued, sleepy, and irritable, not even realizing that these feelings are caused by something in the air, or something in their food or drink, or even something they've touched. They may notice an increase in symptoms, particularly in the eyes, nose, sinuses, or bronchial tubes when they enter a carpeted room, a fabric store, or a new office building. Sometimes symptoms occur when they're exposed to fireplace smoke, paint, gasoline fumes, or car exhaust."

I wished I had a runny nose. *Why does my brain have to swell and cause such bizarre reactions?* I tried to absorb everything Jo was telling me, but very little was really sinking in.

"You don't have to talk," she said, "except to tell me about your symptoms."

I was so grateful for her understanding, I almost started to cry.

"We'll start with a test for formaldehyde. That's in everything from the clothes we wear to the furniture we sit on, even in construction materials used to build houses, stores, and offices," she informed me.

I wondered why more people didn't know about the potentially disastrous effects of everyday chemicals in the environment. Why wasn't the general public more informed about the dangers of toxic exposure? Hosea 4:6 seemed so appropriate: "My people are destroyed from lack of knowledge." The chemical tests made me deathly ill. My heart started pounding and I almost stopped breathing. *Help me, God, please! I can't bear the pain much longer.*

Jo placed me under oxygen for the remainder of the day. "This will help neutralize the symptoms somewhat," she explained. "You'll feel a little better, of course. But we won't be able to get accurate readings on your testing." At that point, I didn't care if they ever completed the tests. I was just grateful for the relief provided by the oxygen.

Jo ran a few more chemical tests the next day, but they continued to make me deathly ill, causing severe tightness in my head and chest. We had to stop for long periods of time between tests, during which I lay on my bed in severe pain and depression. My brain felt like it was going to explode out of my skull.

Well Wishes

Earl and Christie were planning to come see me late Friday afternoon. Greg had gone with a friend to a Texas Rangers baseball game in Arlington. I would miss seeing him, but I was glad he could have some fun and get a little relief from worrying about me. I prayed God would help me recover from the chemical tests so I could have a good visit with my husband and daughter.

When I walked into the visitation area, I saw that Earl and Christie each held an old cardboard shoebox on their lap.

"These are for you, Mom," Christie announced with a broad smile. "I'll read them to you."

Stuffed inside each box were cards and letters from friends as well as from people I had never met, but who had heard about my illness and were praying for me. There must have been more than a hundred cards in those boxes. *Lord, I've experienced some really bad stuff from well-meaning people who are your followers, but Your body is also so beautiful. The love, compassion, and support I'm surrounded with is incredible. Thank you, Jesus, for those who don't understand my illness, but still remain a reflection of your love and compassion.*

We spent most of the evening in the visitation room talking and crying together. Christie sat next to me and held my hand and told me how much she loved me. "I can tell you're doing better today," she said. But I could see the doubt in her eyes as she tried to convince herself.

Poor Earl. I could tell he was exhausted and worried. But he held me and encouraged me, saying, "Everything is going to be okay, Babe."

I told him about the doubts and fears that had been plaguing me.

"Don't worry when you feel like you don't have any faith," he said. "On the day we were married, we became one in God's eyes, so I'll just have faith for you." I thought of Mark 10:7-8 which says, "For this reason a man will leave his father and mother and be united to his wife, and the two become one flesh."

The day went by much too quickly. Earl and Christie stayed in a hotel in Houston that night and promised to be back the next morning. My heart sank again when I watched them leave. Every minute with them was precious to me. Life was precious to me.

I woke up on Saturday very tired and weak. The depression was so heavy I felt completely lifeless and without any shred of hope. *I'm angry, Lord—not really with you . . . well, maybe a little with you. I know you didn't cause this problem in my life, but I know you could take care of it, if you wanted to.*

Nurse Jo came into my room at 10:00 as I laid in bed, staring out the window. "Several of your family members are here to see you," she said in a quiet, soothing voice. "Your brother Hughie, your sister Delores, her husband Sonny. And, of course, Earl, Christie, Greg, and your mom. Which ones would you like to see first?"

"I'm so sick," I moaned, "I don't think I can get out of bed."

"You don't have to see anyone if you don't want to," she offered.

"No," I said, "please send them in." Even if I couldn't muster the energy to make conversation or hide the tears, I could never turn my family away. Jo nodded her understanding and left the room. Moments later, my dad poked his head around the doorway. The sight of him made me weep uncontrollably. He came in and stood next to my bed. I could see he was making a valiant effort to fight back tears.

"Hang in there," he encouraged me, taking my hand. "Everything's going to be okay."

I couldn't even respond. I simply lay there, staring into his sad, misty eyes.

Instead of focusing on my dreadful situation, Dad started to reminisce. He talked about the time he and Greg went fishing at one of the water tanks on our property. "Remember," he said, "we were in that little flat-bottom fishing boat. I leaned over too far to reach for something, and I fell out of the boat into the water. Good thing it was only about four feet deep where we were!" The memory of Dad standing in that water, his hair and face drenched, with that bewildered look in his eyes, made me smile in spite of my pain.

Dad grinned from ear to ear, obviously relieved that he was momentarily able to pull me out of my deep depression with his family story. "When Greg realized I was okay, he started laughing so hard he couldn't stop," he recalled. "There's nothing that boy loves more than getting a good laugh off his PawPaw."

The sadness in Dad's eyes was slowly replaced by joy. It was good to see him look so happy. "Greg's laughing tickled me so much, I started chuckling right along with him," he added.

"Between you splashing in the water and all that laughing," I said, "you guys didn't catch a fish all day." My voice was weak and strained, but I couldn't resist joining in on one of my favorite memories.

"Nope," Dad admitted with a chuckle, "but we sure had a great time."

Throughout the day, Jo brought in various family members and I visited with them all. At the end of the day, I drifted off to sleep with a lighter heart, grateful beyond words for my wonderful, loving family.

Dr. Morlen cut my visiting hours short that night. He had another special test he wanted to perform on me. My brain was so swollen, my body in such severe pain, and my mind so buried in deep depression, that I didn't even listen when he explained what the test was for. I had experienced severe reactions to every single test I had taken, and I had no reason to believe this one would be any different.

I called Earl and informed him of the test.

I followed Dr. Morlen to the testing room like a zombie. Unbelievably, I did not have a single adverse reaction to the test!

Earl called me early the next morning. "I didn't go to bed last night, Babe," he announced.

"Why not?"

"I sat up all through the night and prayed that you would not react to the test." He read 1 Peter 3:7 to me: "You husbands likewise, live with your wives in an understanding way, as with a weaker vessel, since she is a woman; and grant her honor as a fellow heir of the grace of life, so that your prayers may not be hindered" (NAS).

God had certainly answered my husband's prayers! My joy lasted until the first chemical test of the day. The allergen immediately sent me spiraling back into the pits of pain and depression.

Will this cycle never end?

As soon as my reaction began to lessen, another test was administered. There were still several chemicals I needed to be checked for. Time dragged on in an endless stream of torment.

I never want to remember this day again!

Psychologist Visit

I awoke the next morning to unbearable pain and didn't have the emotional or physical energy to do anything. It would be so easy to let myself stop breathing and just die. *God, are you there? Do you care that I'm hurting so badly today? Forgive me, Lord. I can't even begin to imagine your pain on the cross.*

Dr. Morlen said I didn't have to take any more chemical or molds tests—praise God! But that meant I had nothing to do all day except sit and stare out the window, watching, wishing, hoping, and praying for the day I could leave this isolation ward and once again be part of the real world. *Why must I exist when I can't really live?* Life seemed so unfair. I'd lost touch with the outside world. I was detached and disconnected from everyone and everything. *I'm so tired of this place I could scream!*

I tried to trust God completely and not doubt. My mindset was, if I was going to be a strong Christian, my faith should never waiver. But I seemed to have no control over my emotions. *Father, forgive me. I want to love you more, but most of the time I feel nothing except this all-consuming sadness.* Of all the things happening to me, nothing was more painful than the gut-wrenching depression that gripped the very heart and soul of my being. I found comfort in bringing to memory 2 Timothy 2:13: *"If we are faithless, he remains faithful, for he cannot disown himself."*

When I had gone down to the dining room for breakfast, most of the ladies on the unit were sitting together talking. "Linda," Beth said, "We'd love for you to come over here and visit with us." The thought of starting my day hearing all their grueling stories made my stomach churn. Besides, they never talked about how they would get over this illness. Their focus of conversation was always about somehow staying connected as friends because basically their lives were over and they would be in isolation forever, and *my never give up personality wanted no part in that!* I sat alone.

"Linda," Dr. Morlen said after breakfast, "I've made an appointment for you to see Dr. Campbell."

Great. Another doctor.

"She's a psychologist," he added.

"Do you think something is wrong with me because I don't want to constantly hear all their how-I-got-sick stories?"

"Of course not," Dr. Morlen assured me. "But your depression is becoming severe."

No kidding.

"Dr. Campbell will be able to help you cope with your illness."

I didn't want to cope with my illness—I wanted to be cured of it! And I certainly didn't want to speak to a psychologist. I had my pride, after all. But Dr. Morlen didn't care much about my pride.

"I'm afraid I have to insist." He handed me the permission papers that Carolyn had tried to get me to sign on the day I arrived. This time, I seemed to have no choice. I signed, feeling defeated and powerless, with absolutely no control over my own life. Dr. Morlen wasted no time. I was scheduled to see Dr. Campbell that afternoon.

I trudged down the hall to the psychologist's office. I hated that I had to talk to someone I didn't even know and let her tell me how to get a handle on my life. I resented Dr. Morlen for talking me into seeing her. I arrived at the door with Dr. Campbell's name on it and stopped to take a deep breath. *Can't let a shrink see me shaking.* That wouldn't do at all.

I opened the door slowly and peeked inside. The room was plain and simple, just like everything in this unit. Same ceramic tile floor. No pictures on the walls. The computer on the metal desk was encased in stainless steel and vented to keep out the fumes. A metal file cabinet sat next to the metal desk, and beside it was a water cooler with a five-gallon bottle of spring water.

"Hello, Linda," Dr. Campbell greeted me with an outstretched hand. She was about forty years old, tall and slim, with black hair and dark brown eyes. A warm smile lighted her fair complexion, and she spoke with a soft, caring voice. I begrudgingly afforded her an insincere half smile and gave her a limp handshake. Then I slumped into the first available chair. Dr. Campbell seated herself in a matching chair across from me.

"I'm glad you agreed to see me," she began.

"Didn't have much choice," I complained, slouching.

"Dr. Morlen tells me you've been isolating yourself somewhat lately, other than when you're in Bible study. He's quite concerned about you."

"I think he should be more concerned about the rest of the women in this place," I scoffed. "They all seem to enjoy telling their little stories about how they got sick. Everyone around here seems to get a buzz from hearing all the gritty details, but frankly, I get tired of hearing it."

"Maybe you should talk more to others about your story, Linda."

"I refuse to spend my time dwelling on how I got sick. I'd rather search for answers that will set me free from this burden on my life."

"What kind of answers?"

This woman was getting on my nerves. I felt absolutely no compulsion to share my life philosophies with a shrink. If I told her I was trusting God to heal me in a miraculous way, she probably would label me a nut case!

"I really don't want to discuss it, Dr. Campbell."

"Please," she said in a sweet voice, "call me Grace."

I'd just as soon not call you anything. Ever.

"Linda, getting help is not a sign of weakness," Grace assured me.

That touched a nerve. How, after spending such a short time with me, was she able to pinpoint my most basic, underlying fear about this visit?

"Sometimes," she continued, "God uses others to help us when life seems dark and hopeless."

God? Had I heard her correctly?

"Do you," I stuttered, "b-believe in God?"

"Very deeply." Grace smiled. "I accepted Christ as my personal Savior when I was a little girl."

I couldn't recall ever hearing about many Christian psychologists. I'd always thought Christians weren't supposed to seek help from professional counselors. If a believer had a problem, she should simply turn to God for help. If the problem was severe, she could talk to her pastor, or perhaps an older believer. But psychology was based on humanistic philosophies, and psychologists generally tried to convince people that society, or their childhood, or their inner "id" was responsible for all their problems.

Besides that, my deep-seated sense of Dad's family pride and self-sufficiency precluded any thought of seeking help from others, especially a stranger . . . even if she was a believer. I didn't want to share my struggles with her and be analyzed, pigeon holed, and diagnosed with some strange psychological disorder.

"Do you believe in God, Linda?" she asked.

"Yes, but I have really struggled with my faith lately," I admitted. "I know in my heart that God is there, but sometimes in my mind I can't seem to find Him anywhere."

She nodded, a nonverbal encouragement for me to continue.

"So many people have told me that if I have enough faith, God will give me whatever I ask for. They tell me about people getting healings, jobs, houses, even cars, just by believing that God will give those things to them." Now that I had started talking, I couldn't seem to stop. "I don't want money or material things. I just want my life back. I would gladly give up everything I have just to be a normal person again—a wife . . . mother . . . daughter . . . sister . . . friend." I felt my emotions crashing over me in a wave and stopped myself before I completely collapsed.

"How is your family dealing with all that's happened to you?" Grace prodded.

"It's as foreign to them as it is to me," I blurted out. "I can't begin to imagine how confused they must be. I can't even understand this strange illness, and I'm the one who's got it."

"What do you find most confusing?" she asked.

I thought about that for a long moment. So many things about my life were confusing. But one facet did rise to the surface. "The debilitating depression. It's like a monster trying to consume me. It attacks without warning and seems to devour my very soul."

"Desperate feelings are a perfectly normal response to all the losses you've suffered," Grace assured me. "On top of that, your allergic reactions cause your brain to go into a chemical imbalance. That chemical imbalance makes your mind foggy and your emotions unstable."

"So at least some of the depression is the result of my chemical sensitivities?" I found it comforting to know that someone other than the doctors understood the allergic aspect of my depression. It was good to have her confirm that there was a physical explanation to my emotional problems. That meant there could be a tangible cure.

"Absolutely." Grace nodded. "Environmental Illness is physically painful and emotionally embarrassing to begin with. But the disease is also a direct cause of depression. Exposure to allergens results in physiological reactions that cause the brain's chemistry to change, resulting in severe depression."

Now we were getting somewhere. "How can I know when my emotions are real and when they're just the result of allergic reactions taking place in my brain?"

"It's impossible to sort out everything, Linda."

But that was what I wanted. To sort out everything into neat little boxes, that I could compartmentalize and analyze. *Why did life have to be so complex?* Then again, whether the depression was caused by physical or emotional responses, the bottom line was that I hurt . . . beyond anything I had ever thought possible.

"How can I explain to people that my depression is physical, at least in part?" I asked. "Is there anything I can say that will help them understand the physiological aspects of my depression?" The concept of anyone being depressed because their brain chemistry was out of balance due to allergic reactions—and that it's beyond their control to get it back into balance—was beyond comprehension.

"How do other people perceive your struggles with depression?" Grace asked.

"Some people," I explained, "except Earl, Christie, Greg, Mom, Dad, and Earl's mom, of course, seem to think I should be able to control my emotions. They don't understand my depression is the result of a chemical imbalance in my brain resulting from the gas leak in our home that over-powered my immune system."

"What's it like for you, not being understood?"

"It's incredibly frustrating. It hurts. Deeply."

"In what way?" she delved.

"I feel like my personal integrity has been lost. I'm in a constant battle to defend myself. It's exhausting, maddening, and beyond humiliation. And it's a battle I can never win. The only possible outcome seems to be total defeat."

"Do you have any Christian friends who might understand?"

"Yes, but a few of them told me that my depression, like my disease, is spiritual in nature. They say that if I confess my sins and have unshakable faith, I should never be bothered by any sickness or depression."

"How do you feel about that?"

"Exhausted," I cried. "My body and my mind are so stressed out from trying to receive a healing, it'll be a miracle if I ever get well!"

"Do you feel that there's something you need to do, Linda, something that's keeping you from receiving a healing from God?"

All my frustrations came rushing to the forefront. "I've already con-fessed every sin I can think of."

"Do you understand that once you have confessed a sin, it is forgiven, settled, as if it never happened?"

Yes, I knew that, in my head. But hearing it from her made it begin to seem real.

She continued. "We don't have to become perfect little gods in order to receive healing or any other blessing from the Lord. We just need to trust Him, totally, with our lives."

I was beginning to realize that, for me, trust would have to be a step beyond faith. I could have faith that God had the power to control and change my life, but was I willing to trust Him with whatever He chose to do with it?

"Linda, when you're depressed, don't let anyone tell you it's all about a lack of faith or sin in your life," she reassured me.

Grace opened the Bible that was sitting on a nearby table. She turned to Psalm 139:16 and read, "Your eyes saw my unformed substance, and in Your book all the days of my life were written before ever they took shape, when as yet there was none of them" (AMPC).

Then she assured me, "God has a plan for your life, Linda. Don't ever forget that." She closed the Bible and asked, "Are you familiar with the story of Job?"

"Yes." I had read many times the Old Testament story of a man afflicted with physical disease, the loss of all his children, and a wife who turned her back on God and encouraged him to do the same.

"Remember Job's friends? They tried to tell him that his pain and suffering was the direct result of a lack of faith, or some unconfessed sin in his life."

I'd always thought of Job's friends as cruel and non-empathetic.

"Job's friends were wrong, of course. But they honestly believed, in their hearts, that they were doing the right thing, that they were speaking for Job's benefit."

Complete idiots.

"But Job knew he stood righteous and blameless before God. He didn't let his holier-than-thou friends get the better of him. He stood fast and firm, and he trusted that God would vindicate him in the end."

"I don't think I can be as strong as Job," I said.

Grace encouraged me to surround myself with Christians who believed in me, starting with my family and the ladies I'd met my first day in the hospital. "Get involved with people who will love you and pray for you," she advised, "and stay away from those who discourage you, even when they mean well."

Dr. Campbell prayed with me, squeezing my hand through the whole prayer. I left her office in higher spirits than I'd felt since this strange episode of my life began. As I walked back to my room, I realized getting help wasn't a sign of weakness. Instead it was a sign of strength and courage . . . taking down walls, being vulnerable, and making the choice to share your heart and soul with another human being. The decision to talk with Grace was the beginning of the reshaping and remolding of my view of sharing my God-given emotions. I had a ways to go, but I had to hold on to my belief that God had a plan for my life.

CHAPTER SEVEN

GOING HOME

For I am going to do something in your days that you would
not believe, even if you were told.
—Habakkuk 1:5

ON WEDNESDAY MORNING, Dr. Morlen said the most exciting words I'd heard in weeks.

"Would you like to go home this weekend?"

"You mean, like, for a visit?" My heart began racing wildly.

"No, Linda." He smiled. It was the first time I'd ever seen a look of happiness on his face. "I mean, to live." He had such compassion for his patients. It was as if he could feel our pain and sense of hopelessness.

He told me that the hospital had done all they could do for me. "If your husband can create a safe room, an isolation room, for you, I will let you leave the hospital."

"He'll do it," I assured him. "Whatever it takes." I recalled how I'd balked when the doctor first told me we would have to strip out our entire house. Now I was jumping at the chance, eager to do whatever was necessary to get me out of this place and back with my family.

"Everything has to come out of the room," he reiterated, "the carpet, furniture, clothes, decorations—everything."

"No problem."

"If you stay in your safe room for extended periods of time, your immune system will hopefully improve somewhat because it won't be getting constant exposures to the various things you are allergic to. So you won't be able to leave your safe room and go into other parts of the house—especially not the game room."

It would be difficult to stay in a single room full time, but at least it would be a room in my own home instead of this sterile, lonely hospital ward.

"For at least the first year, you'll have to rotate your diet—you cannot eat the same food more often than once every four days. I usually recommend rotating every seven days, but there aren't enough foods that you can reasonably tolerate to be able to last seven days."

"What happens if I eat something less than four days after the last time I had it?"

"Your body will become hypersensitive to it again. You'll start getting ill every time you eat, so you'll eat less and your weight will start falling off again."

I sure don't need that!

I looked around me at the cold, gray walls I'd grown accustomed to over the previous eighteen days. I looked out my window at the outside world—the world full of dust and pollens and molds and toxic chemicals, and . . . Suddenly, without warning, a stark fear gripped me.

"What will happen . . . out there?" I asked, my voice trembling a bit.

"When a patient leaves this pure environment," he said, "it is not uncommon for their body to react severely to everything. Your reactions will be difficult to tolerate at first."

I couldn't imagine things being any worse than they had been for months. *Father, help me to trust you. I'm so scared of what might happen.* The Lord reminded me of Philippians 4:13: "I can do all things through Him who strengthens me" (NAS).

I called Earl right away. "I have good news and bad news," I began. The good news was that I was coming home. The bad news was that my life was still not going to be normal by any stretch of the imagination. Still, we praised the Lord for His goodness.

Getting to Know Flo

When I returned to my room I looked over at Flo, remembering how I had begged to be taken out of room 449B when I was first admitted to the unit. When I saw Flo that day, I became frightened and wanted to run away. Seeing her had made me feel lifeless and hopeless, as I sensed death's grip tugging on my own life.

But obviously God had a plan for me being in room 449B, because I had been privileged to have many conversations with Flo about Jesus Christ, even though most were more like one-sided monologues. After eighteen days of faithfully reading the Scriptures to her every day, I wondered how much of it had sunk in. It struck me that if I was going to be leaving soon, I had little time left to make an impact on Flo's life.

Breathing a fervent prayer, I approached her bed. The rattles and wheezes of her monitoring equipment no longer frightened me. I grasped Flo's hand and rubbed it. When she looked up at me, her eyes seemed more coherent, more conscious than I had ever seen them.

I asked Flo if she would like me to share with her the essence of the Bible study we'd had. As always, she graciously agreed. When I tried to explain to Flo that nothing except our life after death is eternal and therefore truly significant, I asked her if she knew where she would be for eternity after she left this world. Her eyes began to fill with tears and she shook her head no.

I asked if she would allow me to explain to her how she could forever settle any question she might have about eternity.

This time, she nodded yes.

I breathed another quick prayer, then began to tell Flo about God's plan of salvation.

"Because of your sinful nature, you—like all of us—are lost without Christ." I opened my Bible and read to her Romans 3:23: "For all have sinned and fall short of the glory of God."

"We all deserve a death sentence," I explained. "But God chose to reconcile our sin by sending His Son, Jesus Christ, to live the perfect life God's holiness demands." I turned over a few pages to Romans 6:23, "For the wages of sin is death," I read, not knowing whether any of my words were getting through to Flo, "but the gift of God is eternal life in Christ Jesus our Lord."

"Flo," I asked, "do you understand that you have sin in your life?"

She nodded her head, slowly but perceptively.

"Jesus died on the cross for us," I said with a ray of renewed hope. "For you and me." I flipped back a page. "Romans 5:8 says, "But God demonstrates his love toward us in this: While we were still sinners, Christ died for us."

"Do you know that God loves you, Flo?" I asked.

Tears came into her eyes and she shook her head no. I couldn't imagine what life must be like for someone who didn't know that God loved them.

Then I thought of the many times since my illness that I had felt abandoned and unloved by God. If He had the power of life and death in His hands, why did He allow pain and suffering in people's lives? I knew these same doubts must be plaguing Flo's heart. I whispered a quick prayer, then went on.

"All that God requires of us is to repent of our sins and begin a new life in Christ." I read Romans 10:9: "If you declare with your mouth, 'Jesus is Lord,' and believe in your heart that God raised him from the dead, you will be saved."

A single tear escaped from Flo's eye and started to follow the path of a wrinkle toward her ear. I brushed her face with my fingers. Her cheek felt warm.

Fighting my own tears, I explained to Flo that when God created mankind He knew the world would be filled with evil and sin. He also knew that people would live contrary to God's laws. As a result, man would have to suffer consequences of various kinds.

I'd studied these truths countless times over the years in Sunday school lessons and Bible studies and church services. I believed them with all my heart. But never had it seemed so important to convey them to another human being as it did in that moment. I grasped for just the right words.

I looked into Flo's eyes. Again, I could not tell if my words were getting through to her. But, in faith, I continued. "Flo, even if you are never healed, I want you to know that God loves you. His love for us cannot be judged by the condition of our health or the circumstances of our lives."

"Even though God is able to heal anyone at any time, He works according to His own will and plan. God is Sovereign. If God chooses to heal one person and not another, that doesn't mean He loves the healed person more than one who wasn't healed. We just have to trust Him with the life He has given us, no matter how short or long, no matter how healthy or unhealthy our lives might be."

The Apostle Paul struggled with a "thorn in the flesh" for years. I opened my Bible and read, "Three different times I begged the Lord to take it away. Each time he said, 'My grace is all you need. My power works best in weakness.' So now I am glad to boast about my weaknesses, so that the power of Christ can work through me" (2 Corinthians 12:8–9 NLT).

"Sickness isn't always the result of sin in someone's life. Disease and suffering are part of this fallen and toxic world that we live in."

I thanked God that He had taught me these truths so I could pass them on to this sweet, wonderful woman. In the short time I had been Flo's roommate, I had grown to love her. And I knew God loved her even more. He had known Flo her whole life, more intimately than I—or anyone else—ever could. He created her in her mother's womb and knew every day of her life from the beginning to the end.

"Flo, I'll confess to you, I haven't been happy with this illness and I struggle with being angry at God because my life has fallen apart. I continue to pray for healing. Sometimes it's so hard to comprehend and accept God's Sovereignty."

"But, because of the blood Jesus shed on the cross, if we have accepted Him as Savior one day we all will receive total and complete healing, as well as everlasting life with Him in heaven."

I paused, imagining myself walking around heaven, with the new and completely healthy body God would give me when I arrived. I could see

Flo there, too, young and vibrant and fully alive. We would walk—no, we would run and skip and jump and dance together, praising God with our every breath.

Then I realized that Flo's name was not yet written in the Lamb's Book of Life. Until she accepted Christ, she did not have the assurance I did of spending eternity in heaven with God.

"Flo," I whispered, "just think. Even if you were the only person God chose to create, He would still love you so much He would give His one and only Son, Jesus, to die on the cross for you. And all you have to do to receive forgiveness and eternal life is to ask Him into your heart right now, giving Him authority to become your personal Lord and Savior."

Flo looked directly into my eyes for the first time. I asked her if she would like me to go over the steps to accepting Christ. Without hesitation, she nodded yes.

My pulse quickened as I set down the Bible and took Flo's hands in mine.

"Flo," I said, my words catching in my throat, "do you admit that you have sin in your life that separates you from Jesus Christ?"

She nodded.

"Do you believe that God loves you so much that He sent His only Son, Jesus, to pay for your sin?"

Once again, she indicated yes with a nod.

"Do you understand that no matter what sins you have committed, God loves you, and by simply asking Him to forgive you, He will?"

Flo's lips curled into a beautiful, peaceful smile.

"And that He will separate our sins from us as far as the east is from the west, and He will remember them no more" (Psalm 103:12 NIV).

Flo's smile widened as her lips opened to form the word yes. My heart skipped a beat.

"Flo, do you understand that only Jesus Christ can cleanse you from sin and offer you eternal life?"

Once again her lips formed a silent yes.

"Do you want to ask Jesus into your heart and life right now?"

As I looked into her eyes, she actually whispered, "Yes." It was faint but unmistakable.

"Would you like to pray the prayer of salvation with me?"

"Yes," she whispered again, this time with perfect clarity.

My eyes filled with tears as I took another deep breath. I was humbled to be a small part of God's plan for Flo's eternal life and honored that God had ordained our room assignment.

At my prompting, Flo repeated my words in an audible, but shaky, voice, "Dear God, I thank you for life. I thank you for sacrificing your one and only Son, Jesus Christ, to die on the cross to cleanse me from my sin. Right now I ask you to forgive me for my sins. I choose to trust you, and I accept you as the Savior and Lord of my life."

As Flo and I said "Amen," we let the tears stream down our faces. I wrapped my arms around her shoulders and hugged her, our tears mingling together. I knew, without a shadow of doubt, that I would be spending eternity with this dear, lovely woman.

I woke up the next morning with the same horrible feeling of depression that greeted me every day. I felt alone and isolated—stripped of my dignity and self-worth. I had to remind myself that my depression was the result of an allergic reaction that changed the chemistry of my brain, not sin in my life or me choosing to be depressed. Last night had been so wonderful. I was excited and happy for Flo. Those feelings and emotions were so real — and here I was back in the same pit of depression, also just as real. It was hard for me to believe I could swing back and forth like this when I'd always been so in control of my life and been such a happy, content person. Now this depression was destroying me.

Please, Father, give me peace. I still believe you will heal me, but the wait is so long and unbearable. Please use my time of suffering to reshape me, mold me, and refine me, so I can be of service to you.

I had never known such suffering. There was no escape—none—except my quiet times alone with God.

I sat on my bed, trying to read my Bible, but Flo started mumbling, breaking my concentration. I tried to ignore the noise, but she just got louder. Finally I closed the Bible and walked over to her bed.

She looked up at me with clear eyes. "For God so loved the world," she said, "that he gave his only Son, that whoever believes him shall not perish but have eternal life." She smiled and blinked away a tear, then repeated John 3:16 over and over again.

Flo was still bedridden, continuing to draw closer to death every day. But for the first time since I was brought into this ward, I saw a sense of peace and contentment on her face. Gone was the aura of hopeless defeat that had been evident in her demeanor from the moment I met her.

When the nurse came in with our breakfasts, Flo gave her a great big smile and said, "God loves me." All day long, whenever we were alone in the room, Flo chanted John 3:16. Every time someone came in, Flo told them, "God loves me" and flashed a beautiful, confident smile.

Homeward Bound

On Friday, Earl arrived at the clinic right after lunch. I gathered the few belongings I had brought in with me and anxiously waited for him to take care of all the financial matters. When he finally returned to my room, he asked if I was ready to go. It took only a fraction of a second for me to answer yes.

Those cold metal doors looked a lot better going out than they had going in! My heart raced as the nurse pushed me in a wheelchair down those long corridors of the hospital. I was going home, but to many unknowns and uncertainties.

I began to wonder what it would be like to live isolated in my own home. *What would my bedroom look like?*

Earl hooked me up to a cylinder of oxygen that he had purchased to use on the trip, as well as in my "safe room" after I returned home. I was so weak and frail, he and the nurse had to lift me into the front seat of the car. Earl wanted me close to him in case I suddenly became ill on the long drive home. He was worried about me reacting to the exhaust from cars, pollens, and everything else.

The drive was grueling. I felt deathly ill.

"We're gonna get you home, Babe," Earl assured me. "Try to hang in there. You'll be better once we get you home."

The scenery outside the car window sped by faster and faster as Earl tried to make the long drive as short as possible.

"Oh, no," he groaned as a patrolman's siren and spinning lights forced him to pull over. The officer approached Earl's window, which he reluctantly rolled down.

"You were driving awfully fast there, sir," the patrolman pointed out the obvious. "You got some kind of emergency there?" He glanced at me, and his expression changed completely. "Guess you do," he mumbled, and didn't say another word about speeding. I must have looked like I was on my death bed. "Just be as careful as you can," he advised, returning to his vehicle without even asking for Earl's driver's license. We quickly got back on the road again to complete our trip.

As we entered the city limits of Brownwood, I laid down on the car seat. Pride consumed me. I didn't want anyone to see me.

But when I felt the car rumble across a cattle guard, I sat straight up. That cattle guard meant we were crossing onto our property. I knew I was as safe as I could be. I was finally home with my family, who loved me and would protect me to the best of their ability.

I stared out the car window, unable to hold back the tears. Home had never looked so wonderful. My tears came from both joy and sadness. I was thrilled to be back with my family, of course, but fearful of what it would be like to live in isolation. Mostly, I was just glad to be home.

Earl's mother, Grandmother, stood on the front porch, waving so hard I thought her arm would fall off.

"Christie's at her volleyball game," Earl explained, "and your mom and Greg went to Pearland for the weekend." Mom had been staying at our home in Brownwood to take care of Earl and the kids and to be able to visit me while I was in the hospital. Dad had stayed home in Pearland. He was recently retired, but worked for my brother Hughie running errands, ordering materials, and doing various odd jobs for his security systems business. He also had a garden going year round, so he couldn't be away from home for long periods of time.

"Your dad's birthday was yesterday," Earl explained, "so your mom and Greg went to Pearland to celebrate with him."

I had missed my father's birthday. I felt terrible for not even remembering his special day.

"Your mom knew she wouldn't be able to get back home for a while once you got here. After we get you all set up, she'll be pretty busy taking care of you," Earl explained. "School will be starting in a few weeks, so she'll be helping get the kids to all their school activities. This will probably be Greg's only chance to visit with his PawPaw for a while. He'll be awful busy once school starts up."

We pulled into the driveway and my heart began to race. I attempted to prepare myself for the changes that had taken place in our home, especially in my bedroom.

Earl helped me get out of the car and placed my oxygen tank next to me. I attempted to make my own way up the sidewalk, pulling the tank on wheels. But I was weak and very unstable. When Earl saw me faltering, he quickly came to my rescue and steadied me.

I headed slowly for the front door. In the past, I usually went in the side door through the game room. But that room still had high levels of chemicals in it. As I passed that side door, a deep sadness swept over me. I remembered all the plans and dreams we had had when we chose to build the room—lots of fellowships for young people, fun times with people our age, family gatherings. I got teary eyed and quickly looked in the opposite direction.

When I neared the front porch, I stood there for a few minutes and looked out over our land. I remembered the last time I had done this, when I gazed at the sunrise out the laundry room window thinking, "My life is so perfect." I remembered, too, that voice—that evil voice warning me that I was going to have to die.

I hadn't died. But my life had certainly become scary and difficult.

Grandmother greeted me with a hug and a kiss on the cheek. She and I had always spent a lot of time together shopping or working on projects. She told me how glad she was that I was home and that she would be so happy to take care of me.

When I entered the living area, I stopped and stared at the strange-looking room. The walls were bare. No decorations of any kind graced the sparse furniture. All the lovely paintings and family photographs had disappeared. The certificates of accomplishment we had all received over the years, which I had carefully framed and hung . . . all were gone. Earl's and my college degrees. All of Christie and Greg's academic awards and trophies. The room looked as if a thief had come in and stolen everything—things that had far more sentimental value than monetary worth. Even my beautiful silk flower arrangements were noticeably missing.

"I removed all the plastic articles in the kitchen," Grandmother explained as we walked slowly down the hall toward my bedroom. "I got rid of all the cleaning supplies, and the scented soaps and shampoos from the bathrooms and dressing areas."

Everywhere I looked, I noticed things that I had taken away from my family. Feelings of guilt and sadness threatened to overwhelm me.

Further down the hall, we passed by the children's rooms. I peeked through the open doorways. The rooms looked stark and bare, cleared of all the many things that might cause me to react. Christie's room was void of perfume, makeup, and nail polish . . . all the things a young girl enjoyed. Greg's room had lost all the car models he had so painstakingly put together. His Star Wars figures were gone, too . . . probably tucked away behind his closed closet door.

I finally reached my bedroom in the back part of the house. Through the closed door, I heard the annoying hum of the air purifier Earl had purchased for me, based on Dr. Morlen's recommendation. It sounded exactly like the ones I'd grown sickeningly accustomed to in the hospital.

I knew how expensive those air purifiers were. And I knew our insurance would not cover any of the cost. But we had no other choice.

Grandmother opened the door and I stood there in shock. My once-beautiful, cozy bedroom had become cold and sterile, stripped of everything warm and inviting. The plush brown-and-gold carpet and padding had been ripped out, leaving just a cold concrete-slab floor. Gone were my lovely, custom-made ivory curtains with the blue trim, leaving the windows bare and exposed.

The only furniture in the room was two cots—one for me and one for Earl. They were aluminum, with pillows and blankets of a plain, natural color. A cylinder of oxygen perched on a stand next to one cot.

Earl helped me sit down on the cot. "Look what I got for you," he said, picking up a glass-and-steel box that had been sitting on the other cot. "I bought one of those reading boxes for you, like Dr. Morlen told us about. One of his patients in Houston had a mild case of Environmental Illness. She no longer needed it, so I bought it from her."

Lucky her.

"I picked up these pillows and blankets from the store in the allergy clinic. They're made of 100 percent organic cotton, of course. I got a mold testing kit, too. That place has all kinds of environmentally healthy products. And they have a huge selection of spring waters all bottled in glass, instead of plastic."

How exciting.

Earl pointed toward the door to my connecting bathroom. "We replaced your soap, shampoo, and cream rinse with unscented brands, and got you some baking-soda deodorant and toothpaste. Grandmother and your Mom went shopping and found you some plain white cotton clothes. We took all the polyester and colored stuff out of your closet so it wouldn't bother you."

I appreciated all the effort my family had gone through for me. And I was grateful to finally be home. But I wondered how I would ever be able to live like this.

"And I found this phone you can use." I stared at the old telephone sitting on the floor beside my cot. "It shouldn't have any more plastic smell since it's been around so long, so hopefully it won't cause you any problems."

I lay down on the cot and closed my eyes. Earl and Grandmother sensed I needed some time alone and left the room, closing the door softly.

Stark and Sterile

It was good to be home, but I felt a familiar and overwhelming sense of guilt as I thought about all the changes that had taken place in my family's lives because of me.

Maybe it would be better for everyone if I'd just stayed in the hospital in Houston. If I wasn't at home, my family wouldn't have to be constantly aware of my bizarre illness and all it had taken from them.

I was again assaulted with the morbid thought that it might be best for my family if I just died. I remembered the strong urge I'd had the day Earl took me to the hospital and I wanted to start running and never stop. Once again, I wanted to run, to search for a "safe place." As my mind started racing, searching for the Lord, the Holy Spirit spoke to my heart and reminded me of the verse that had become my life motto. "For I know the plans I have for you." I thanked God for His faithfulness to me and to His Word and His promises.

Then I recalled the cruel voice that had said, "You're going to have to die. You're going to have to die." My battle was still raging, but God was in control of my life. I knew I must trust Him with every fiber of my soul.

I opened my eyes and looked around at my cold, stark room. I gazed at the closed door, a powerful reminder of how closed off I still was to the outside world. Near the door was a long, high window about two feet wide. On the other side of that window was the game room.

I dragged myself off my cot and slowly crossed the room. With mixed emotions, I slowly drew back the mini-blinds. They were several years old, so they wouldn't emit any fumes I might be allergic to.

I peeked through the glass and stared at the game room. There sat the jukebox, dark and quiet. The pool and ping pong tables still looked brand new, as if they'd never been used. The big-screen TV looked strange to me without a stainless steel case to vent the fumes, like the ones in the hospital. The built-in shelves still held rows of old classic movies, exercise programs, and home videos . . . none of which I was able to view. The walls still boasted portraits of the children. My family was not even allowed to go into this room anymore. Earl told me he'd sealed off the entrance with large tarps so the toxic fumes couldn't escape into the hallway and make their way into my room.

Symptoms and Realities

I napped in the afternoon. That evening Earl woke me up to give me my allergy shots and to feed me some supper. I nibbled at the baked turkey and black-eyed peas. But after just a few bites, I began to experience shortness of breath and felt like I was going to pass out. Earl took the nearly untouched tray back to the kitchen. Within a few minutes my symptoms started to settle down.

Grandmother came in to let me know she was going to her house for a while. "Do you need anything, Hon?"

I could think of lots of things I needed. My life. My health. Pain medication that wouldn't make me sick. There was nothing that she, or anyone, could provide. I shook my head, and she left my room.

I decided to take a shower, hoping it would help me feel better, both physically and emotionally. Earl had a water purification system installed in the house to remove the chlorine that I was so desperately allergic to. When I entered my dressing room, my reflection in the mirrored cabinets caught my attention. I stopped and stared. Could that sickly, frail woman in the mirror possibly be me? I looked like a ghost, all thin and pale. The mirrors ran the length of the sinks and dressing table that connected my bedroom to the bathroom. There was no way I could avoid seeing myself several times a day, every day.

Focusing on the wall opposite the mirrors, I proceeded to the shower. The unscented shampoo and cream rinse left my hair tangled, lifeless, and feeling like straw, but at least it was clean. I missed the fresh herbal scent of my regular shampoo. I missed the sweet-smelling body lotion I used to put on after every shower. I couldn't even rub lotion into my dry hands. And the special treat of a long, soothing bubble bath was a thing of the past.

I braved a look at myself in the mirror as I dragged an old comb through my wet hair. You could really use some makeup, girl, I told my reflection. I pulled open the mirrored door of my medicine cabinet. The shelves were empty. All my makeup was gone.

I opened a drawer. No more curling iron or hot rollers. Not even a blow dryer. I slammed the drawer closed and stared into the mirror again. My wet hair hung limp around my shoulders. With a shrug of resignation, I returned to my cot, laid my damp head on the white cotton pillow, and slipped into a temporary state of sweet unconsciousness.

When I awoke the next morning, the first thing I saw was Earl sleeping on the cot next to me. I was so glad to be home! But I was also weak and tired, and Earl had to help me sit up on the side of my cot and then assist me in walking around. It was a major challenge just to stand up, an even greater hurdle to take a few steps. After just a few minutes, I asked him to let me lie down and rest.

After helping me back to bed, he said "I'm going to go to the kitchen now and get you some breakfast." He brought back a tray with two bowls of plain oatmeal and two glasses of spring water.

"You don't have to eat this just because I do," I told Earl. "You should eat normal food."

"Don't want to," he said, stirring his hot oatmeal with a spoon. "When we eat together, I'll have whatever you're having."

"Don't be ridiculous," I complained.

"And I won't have anybody else eating in front of you, either." He slipped a big spoonful of oatmeal into his mouth.

"I appreciate how much you want to protect me," I said, staring at the steaming mush. How could I explain to him that I just wanted to protect everyone else. "But I want my life to be as normal as possible. I don't want to take anything else away from my family, and that includes food."

Earl just smiled and continued eating. Reluctantly, I tried a bite of the bland breakfast. I noticed it was flavored with a tiny bit of salt. I missed the fresh fruit, butter, milk, and pure maple syrup that used to drench our oatmeal.

"Where are Christie and Grandmother?" I asked. "I'd like to see them."

"It's Sunday, Babe," Earl reminded me. "They went to church."

It hurt so much not to be able to attend services with my family.

"You should have gone with them," I said, "instead of staying home with me."

"No way," he chided me with a smile. "I'm going to be your constant bodyguard."

On Sunday evening when Greg and Mom returned home from Pearland, they came directly to my bedroom. I could hear them through the closed door as soon as they neared my room. Mom started hugging me with tears flowing down her cheeks. "Baby," she kept saying, "I never stop praying that God will heal you. You don't worry about a thing. Grandmother and I will take care of everything."

As soon as Mom let go of me, Greg came over with a big smile on his face and hugged me. "I'm so glad you're home," he said. He told me all about his trip to Mom's house and how much fun he'd had hanging out with "PawPaw."

Monday morning I woke up sick and couldn't talk or even lift my head off the pillow. Earl had to return to work, and I hated thinking about it. I would miss his constant love and support. After he had eaten breakfast, Earl came back into our bedroom to tell me good-bye. Kneeling beside my cot he said, "I wish I didn't have to leave you, Babe." He looked distraught.

"I wish that too," I said. "But we don't have any choice. You have to go to work."

With tears in his eyes, he told me he would be praying for me all day. "And if you need me, just have your mom or Grandmother call and I'll come right home."

He kissed me and hugged me. We said a prayer together and I held onto him as long as I could.

"I'll be back at lunchtime to give you your noon injections," he promised.

The minute he walked out the door I experienced an overwhelming feeling of aloneness. Mom and Grandmother would be there all day, checking on me. I was very appreciative of them, but they could not fill the void that only Earl could. And yet, I knew that if something happened to me, one way or the other Earl would take care of me like he had always done.

I looked at my watch throughout the long morning, counting the moments until lunchtime. About fifteen minutes before noon, Earl came through my bedroom door. I felt safe again the second his face appeared. The hour passed by much too quickly. Earl gave me my injections, we talked for a few minutes, then he went into the breakfast room to eat a quick bite of lunch. He came back with a plate of baked chicken, green beans, and an orange. While I ate, we talked and shared Scripture verses with each other. Then we prayed together.

When Earl told me he had to go back to the office, my heart sank once again. I hated to see him leave. I watched the clock all afternoon until he came home. Lying on my cot and staring out the bedroom window, I fought the tormenting depression and wished I would wake up from this hellish nightmare.

"Lord, do you realize I have been going through this ordeal for five months? I can't take this isolation, pain, helplessness, and depression any longer."

I felt and heard no response.

I sat up on the side of my cot looking outside at the world I could no longer be a part of. Crying from the bottom of my heart and soul, I buried my face into my trembling hands and I sought God once more.

Father God, how can you allow your children to suffer? I'd never stand by and watch my children suffer like this if I had the power to change things. I don't understand suffering . . . and I don't like it.

Still no response!

God, I have been warring with this 'dance of death' way too long. I'm weak. I have to constantly fight the enemy who wants me to give up. Sometimes I'm tempted. What have I done to deserve this? I want my life back, please.

Silence.

Greg and Christie came in to check on me. After a long, silent look, they left the room with tears in their eyes. I heard Christie's bedroom door close. I was sure I heard her crying, like she seemed to do so often.

A few moments later, Greg came back holding a cotton ball in one hand and a small glass bottle of cooking oil in the other. He approached my bed and knelt beside me. I watched him saturate the cotton ball as tears welled up in his eyes.

"Mom," he said, "I read in the Bible that when someone is sick, you're supposed to anoint their head with oil. We have organic almond oil, and since you eat almonds I thought you'd be okay if I used it."

"I would love that" I said.

Greg whispered an earnest prayer for God to deliver me, then silently touched my forehead with the oil-soaked cotton.

I lay there, tears flowing down my cheeks. Greg wiped my tears and said, "Mom, I know Jesus is going to heal you. I just know it."

What incredible faith for a twelve-year-old boy!

I was overwhelmed with emotion and couldn't speak. I knew if I said anything, it would break a dam of tears and flood the room. I didn't want to take away from what Greg was doing and quickly thought about Mark 10:15, which tells us we can come to the Lord in simple, childlike faith. "Truly I tell you, anyone who will not receive the kingdom of God like a little child will never enter it." I felt God trying to teach me to just relax and rest in Him. He wanted me to have that childlike faith, rather than almost destroying myself and my relationship with Him through my attempts to heal myself.

"Thank you for your prayer," I said to Greg, "and for loving me in all of my brokenness." I told him, again, that I was sorry for making him so sad and for disrupting his life. "And I'm sorry I can't really be much of a mom to you and Christie right now." I saw a worried look cross his face. Never wanting to do anything that would increase my children's distress, I added, "Someday I will be."

"Mom," he said, "I will always love you, no matter what. And you're still the best mom in the world." As he spoke he wiped tears from his eyes and hugged me for a long time.

I felt so inadequate hearing those words. Before this strange disease, my children had rarely seen me cry. I always tried to protect their hearts. But now, they saw my pain every day. I knew I would never forget the sad looks on their faces every time they came to see me.

Later that day, Christie came back and sat with me for a long time. She didn't say or do anything in particular. But her tenderness spoke volumes to me. Her gentle presence made her love and support for me tangible.

Finally, Earl arrived home from work. The second I saw his face, I felt safe again.

God Promises Healing

That night I was suddenly awakened out of a deep sleep. It was pitch black. I sat up and looked around the room. I saw no one, yet was very aware of a presence in the room. Earl was sleeping peacefully on his cot next to mine.

Suddenly, I heard a powerful yet loving voice say, "Behold, I am the Lord thy God that healeth thee. Is there anything too hard for me?"

My heart started to pound. There was something so powerful, so distinct, about the voice that, for the first time, I knew without a doubt that God would restore my health at His appointed time . . . emphasis on "appointed" time, because I would learn the hard way that this difficult journey was far from over.

"At the appointed time I will return to you," concluded the voice.

In that moment I was filled with a renewed sense of hope. I believed beyond a doubt that God would restore my health at His appointed time.

The next morning I couldn't wait to tell my family about the word God had spoken to me.

Earl came in first.

"Babe, I started to wake you up during the night to tell you something. I didn't because I knew how much you needed sleep."

"Tell me about it," urged Earl.

"Well, I was sound asleep and I woke up out of nowhere. Jesus spoke to me. Babe, I heard Him and I felt Him in the room with me."

"What did He say?"

"He said that He would heal me!"

Earl grabbed and hugged me like he had never had before. The love in his embrace assured me there was absolutely no doubt that he believed I had heard from the Lord and could believe He would restore my life. We were still excitedly talking and rejoicing when Mom, Christie, Greg, and Grandmother came in the room to see what the commotion was about.

Greg asked, "What are y'all so excited about? I could hear you talking down the hall from my room."

I replied, "I've heard from the Lord and He is going to heal me."

My account of my visit with my Heavenly Father elated each of them, and they joined in the celebration. My family's faith was strengthened and we eagerly anticipated the day that my health would be renewed, recalling Romans 4:21: "Being fully persuaded that God had the power to do what he had promised."

We began talking about the family trips we would take when I could travel again. Knowing school would be starting soon, my children had thoughts about their hopes and dreams of their future school days.

"I'll just be glad when you can pick us up from school again," Greg said.

"I can't wait till you can come to our school activities," Christie added.

Earl said he looked forward to the day when we could all go to church together again.

We were all encouraged but my battle with depression and a host of other symptoms continued to ravish my mind and body.

CHAPTER EIGHT

VISIONS

I will pour out my Spirit on all people. Your sons and
daughters will prophesy, your old men will dream dreams,
your young men will see visions.
—Joel 2:28

I HAD ALWAYS WORKED HARD to be available for my children. I especially looked forward to the annual back-to-school activities. But this year I could not do anything for my children or go anywhere with them. I was weak— mentally, emotionally, physically, and spiritually. I couldn't be in the same room with their new school supplies or new clothes. I couldn't write their names on anything because of the chemical smell of the felt-tip markers.

Finally, that dreaded day arrived—the first day of the new school year. This would not be the same joyous occasion our family had always experienced. Picking up friends along the way to school and rushing after work to pick everyone up were part of the family traditions that would not take place this year. Instead, I would be left home all day, counting the hours until my children returned home from school. My heart ached.

Unable to return to my job as school nurse, I felt powerful resentment that my career was over. I knew someone had replaced me at the school. Only through the grace of God did I manage to hold back the tears until Mom and the children left the house. Then disappointment and anger engulfed me and I wept bitterly.

"God I don't get it. Why do I continue to be punished by you?" The questions continued to spew out of my mouth. "As school nurse I took care of children whose parents abused and neglected them. And so many times, they were never punished and were allowed to remain a part of their children's lives."

The heart wrenching weeping continued.

"Sometimes I feel you don't love me. I feel so abandoned and alone."

I still couldn't believe my whole world had been snatched from me. I wanted to flee to a secret hiding place, but I could not find such a place. I laid on the cold, hard floor and cried out to the Lord, "God, do you love me?"

The most debilitating reaction to things I was allergic to was depression. Allergies controlled my moods and emotions. Some days I was filled with hope, then others days I felt detached from life and people, and abandoned by God. Most of my time was spent lying on my aluminum cot and crying. "Lord, some days I just wished I were dead. At least in death there would be no pain."

I sat up, took a deep breath, and stared out the window. I was just wishing that I could get back to living life.

"God, how could you love me and allow this to happen to me?"

Suddenly I found myself scanning the bare walls and floors of my bedroom that were as empty and void as my life.

God, I feel somewhat like Job. So many things in my life that I love . . . being a wife, being with and taking care of my children and others, and taking an active role in life, no longer exist.

I walked into my dressing room and washed my face. As I stared into the vanity mirror, my thoughts continued to question the Lord.

How could you love me and allow this to happen? God, are you still there?

I walked back into the bedroom and got on my knees by the aluminum cot that had replaced my beautiful dark brown oak bed.

"Lord," I cried out, "It is so unfair that I push so hard to be happy, to have hope, to believe this terror will end, and a single allergen exposure changes the chemistry of my brain and I'm beneath the pits of Hell with depression. I feel so powerless. How can I change what's happening in my brain? I feel I have no control over my life. I can't control the environment of the world. Please help me."

Why do I have to exist in a world I can't be a part of?

My friends tried to support me, but it wasn't easy. There were so many restrictions that had to be met before they could visit, so my interactions with the outside world were few and far between. God was hearing me, even though I didn't think He cared. One day, He sent me a special friend, Dr. Rainey, a professor at our local university.

Dr. Rainey sent me a note: *Linda, I've never met you but I want you to know that my wife and I have been praying for you. We've heard how difficult this illness has been for your family.*

Friends from our Sunday school class had told me about this person. He was an incredible man of faith, humility, and integrity, they said, filled with wisdom and discernment.

Dr. Rainey's note also announced that the Lord had given him a scripture to share with me. It was Jeremiah 29:11: "For I know the plans I have for you, declares the Lord, plans to prosper you and not to harm you, plans to give you hope and a future."

I was thankful for the uplifting verse and praised the Lord for the confirmation. I was encouraged.

The note continued, *I feel God has instructed me to come to your home and minister to your family by praying for each of you, if that might be possible.*

I responded to Dr. Rainey's note and accepted his offer with deep gratitude. I carefully explained the visitation requirements and set up an evening visit so that Dr. Rainey could come to our home and meet the four of us in my isolation room.

His arrival was refreshing. We talked about faith, miracles, and prayer. Then he went on to explain the process of grief and how each of us was experiencing it in our own way. Before leaving he prayed a powerful prayer over our family. His words and prayer brought comfort and understanding. He assured me that he and his wife, Sue, who was an intercessor, would be praying for me and the family. After visiting for about an hour he bid us farewell, telling me that he would be in contact real soon.

That evening after Dr. Rainey left, I laid on my cot and thought on the words he had spoken to Christie and Greg. "Your mother has not died, yet you have lost her in so many ways. That's why it hurts so badly. You are going through the grieving process now, much like someone experiences when a death occurs." His words made such sense. Death described my life so well—a living death sentence.

A Tribute to Earl

Most of my worldly support and strength came from Earl. He spent every minute he could at my bedside. When I couldn't pray, he prayed for me. When I had no faith, he had faith for me. When I wanted to die, he wouldn't let me. I felt so worthless, but somehow he always managed to prove to me that he valued me far beyond my understanding.

I worried a lot about Earl's level of stress. As much as he possibly could, he chose to take care of me rather than giving the responsibility to his mom and my mom. I knew the main reason was simply his love for me, but I believed it also gave him some sense of control over our lives. Like me, he felt pretty helpless and powerless over my situation.

Earl looked extremely tired and stressed most of the time. The enemy used even this to make me more miserable. He assaulted me with a pervading fear that Earl would die and I would be left alone, without my husband's physical and emotional support, upon which I was so dependent.

One night when Earl came home from work, I told him I wanted him to get me my wedding ring. I'd missed it so much since I took it off when I entered the hospital. I could live without my other jewelry, but my finger felt naked and lost without the symbol of my blessed marriage. I had lost so much weight I barely could keep it on my hand. When Earl slipped my wedding ring onto my left hand, I felt a sense of gratefulness and thought back to the ladies in the Houston hospital whose husbands had walked away from them. I fought to hold back tears.

The next day we had prayed before Earl left for work, and then he slipped his wedding band on my finger. Barely holding back his tears, he whispered, "Today, every time you look at this ring, know that I love you and I'm thinking of you and I'm praying for you."

Huge Inner Battle With God

My days continued to be filled with pain, severe depression, hopelessness, and fear. *What is wrong with me? Why can't I regain control of my life?* Suddenly I realized that I was powerless outside of God. I began to better understand that the only power I could ever have would be that which came through Him.

I finally accepted the fact that the only healing that would ever be mine would come by direct intervention of the great Jehovah Rapha. I needed to better understand His power and diligently searched the scriptures while God was leading me to the truth. I needed to know Him like I'd never known Him before. I needed the mind of Christ to guide me, to teach me. I needed a major God-connect. As I constantly read the Word, I began to better understand the Holy Spirit was my connection with God. It was God's power working in me.

My own willpower that I had always relied on to make things happen wasn't working. Looking back, I realized that by relying on my own power,

I was saying to God, "I don't need you. I can't trust that you are enough to meet my needs."

I knew I had to transform my heart and my thinking. I had to see God was the only power source that would change my life. One day I came across the scripture Romans 12:2: "But be transformed by the renewing of your mind." I knew that I had to do this. I understood renewing my mind would be a process and that fear and unbelief would limit God's working power in my life. I knew I received the Holy Spirit when I received Christ; now I had to give Him permission to perform His will and His power in my life.

I began to ask God, on a daily basis, to speak to me, to reveal Himself to me in His Word or any other way He chose. I lived in a nearly constant state of prayer, seeking the Lord's help and guidance moment by moment. Every day He faithfully honored my request. His answers came mostly in the form of quiet, calm assurance and peace, especially when I was all alone in my room. At other times He spoke to me through the encouraging words of family, friends, or even strangers who had heard about my condition and been prompted by the Holy Spirit to contact me.

But I wanted more. I begged God every day to provide me with some kind of sign that He was still there, that He still cared about me, because depression was always threatening to overtake me. Satan was always ready to attack, whispering in my ear, "God doesn't care." During this torment I didn't know how to take on the spiritual warfare.

As I pondered Satan's words, I became frightened.

But what was I really afraid of? What was at the root of my fear of totally giving control of my life to Christ? Once again, I was afraid of marring my family belief that asking for help was a sign of weakness. What if God asks me to completely change the person I am? I know how to be me, but not how to be someone else. Was He asking me to die to my old self? To become selfless and weak?

My mind continued to search for answers. Was I struggling with pride versus humility? Did I covet my will and pride, when in fact I needed to walk in humility, immersed in God's will? What if He healed me then asked me to share my story? That thought scared me terribly, because no one understood my strange disease. Would people judge me, mock me, walk away from me? I couldn't stand the humiliation and judgmental attitude. Was I unable to give up control because I had formed a barrier around my heart? I didn't want anyone to know how much I was struggling and how weak and powerless I felt.

I wanted to know that one day I would be healed and could return to a normal life. As I prayed, the Lord spoke the same words to me over and over: "Linda, I want you to totally relinquish your life to me."

What if total relinquishment meant that, for the rest of my life, I would have to depend on others to take care of me? I was a nurse. I was supposed to take care of others. I didn't want anyone to have to care for me. That thought was terrifying.

What if total relinquishment involved giving Him my children? That thought terrified me. My immediate thought was, *He can have everything that I have, but I can't relinquish my children to Him. What will He do with them? I'm their mother. No one can love them and care for them like I can. He's God. . . . But I'm their mother. I refuse to give them up!* I'd rather die or remain ill for the rest of my life before making Christie and Greg a sacrifice for my healing.

Surrender

One night after Earl came home from work, he poked his head into my room and announced, "I bought something for you today." Opening the door wider, he walked in carrying a stack of cassette tapes. "This is the entire New Testament," he said, carefully placing the stack on the floor across the room. He then brought in an old cassette player. "This shouldn't bother you because the plastic doesn't smell anymore." He tore the wrapping off the first tape and popped it into the player. "Your mom and Grandmother will have to put the cassettes in for you, since the tapes are new."

I didn't mind. I was just thrilled to have the Word on tape! I could read in my glass box for short periods of time, but some days I was so tired that my eyes wouldn't focus. Earl pushed the Play button. "The book of the genealogy of Jesus Christ, the son of David, the son of Abraham," a rich baritone voice spoke.

I called my husband over and gave him a big hug, thanking him profusely. From that day on I inhaled and digested every word on those tapes. The more I listened, the more I realized that no one can truly understand God's power and love without hearing His Word. I also came to realize that the fullness of His presence in my life was more important than my physical healing.

"Lord," I prayed, "change me into the person you want me to be. I can't do this on my own, but I'm willing to allow you to transform me according to Your will."

Are you? He seemed to ask. *Are you really willing to allow my will, no matter what?*

I sensed the Lord wanted me to totally relinquish control of everything in my life. Again, thoughts of my children came to mind and I couldn't think of anything more difficult for Him to ask of me.

Maybe I felt I had to hold on to what little part of my life I still had control of . . . the right to choose to surrender or the right to continue the fight to survive on my own.

On Wednesday my friend Kathy Rodgers came over to read the Word and pray with me. She stayed for several hours. When Earl came in to give me my shots, she left the room to give us some privacy, but then came right back in. We had a wonderful time together in the Lord.

"I'm going to come here every Wednesday," she promised. From that point on, my faithful friend never missed a single week.

The following Friday evening, Christie came into my room looking sad, obviously fighting back tears. I reached out to hug her, and she fell into my embrace. I didn't say a word because my own tears would flow if I did.

"Mom, God doesn't love me," she said.

"Baby," I said, stroking her hair and looking into her eyes, "what do you mean? Of course God loves you."

"Don't tell me that. If He did, you would be well. And you're not."

I couldn't think of anything to say to my precious daughter. The doubts she expressed were the same ones that had plagued me so often over the past year.

After a few more moments of sobbing, Christie finally explained what had happened. "Today at my volleyball game, as I was on the court playing, I kept staring into the stands. Somehow I knew you would be there. Coach Kennedy kept yelling at me, telling me to get my head in the game. But I couldn't. All I could do was look for you. You'd always been there."

Nothing would have thrilled me more than seeing my daughter's first game of the season. I had never missed any of my children's activities, and it was one of the things that devastated me most.

"Baby, you know I can't —"

She stood abruptly. "You were supposed to be healed by now," she cried. "I've prayed and prayed and prayed."

Christie certainly wasn't the only one.

"I just don't believe God loves me anymore. If He did, He would have healed you by now."

My heart broke to hear Christie say such words. The last thing I wanted was for her to lose her faith in God. But how many times had I entertained those doubts myself?

"I just want to take my fist and beat these walls down and let you out of this room," Christie cried. "It's not fair that you have to live in isolation. It's not fair that you're sick. I hate it!"

A tear slipped down my cheek. "I hate it too," I whispered.

Christie collapsed back into my arms.

I took a deep breath, then did my best to reassure Christie that God would heal me in His way and in His time. I didn't want to mislead her and possibly harm her faith in the Lord further if I wasn't healed physically, completely, or immediately.

Finally, somewhat reassured, Christie's tears ebbed, and so did mine. We prayed together, and the Spirit of God enveloped us both with His peace . . . a peace that certainly did surpass our circumstances! Christie prayed that she would be able to focus on her games, her schoolwork, and everything else that God had called her to do as we waited, together, for His promises to be fulfilled.

As she left and went back to her room, I continued to pray for my sweet, sensitive daughter. *This illness has caused me to doubt my own faith, Lord. I can only begin to imagine how hard this must be for my children!* Each time that I look into their tear filled eyes, I try to comprehend what it must be like to live in the constant fear that their mother might die. I cried as my son and daughter prayed over me with words that were filled with such heart-wrenching pain. They were begging for my healing and asking God to please not let me die. *Please, Father, hold them close to you. Don't let this, or anything else, pull them away from you. You are our only hope!*

Consumed with guilt and fear that I might, through this illness, cause my children to doubt and possibly walk away from their faith, I was desperate to hear from the Lord. I needed to know that He would remain faithful to keep His promises to me. I once again frantically begged Him for confirmation that I would be well again.

"Jesus, please hear my heart-filled prayer. Our family desperately needs to know that you will be faithful to your promises of healing in my life. I am so afraid Christie and Greg's faith will be shattered if they don't soon see evidence of your faithfulness."

As I sat in silence, I heard His gentle voice say, "Linda, faith is my gift given to you through grace. Once I have given you a promise, you will freely receive it through your faith in me . . . not of yourself. Please choose to trust Me."

I felt reassured and comforted by His words. I knew I had to believe that His promises would be guaranteed and delivered no matter what the circumstances were around me.

Because my allergic reactions caused my brain to swell, resulting in confusion, depression, and the inability to think clearly at times, I would doubt my faith. I hated those times. My heart told me one thing, but my emotions told me something so differently. During these moments, I battled to keep believing what I knew deep inside was true. God would be faithful. I was learning to trust my heart and not my emotions. I begged the Father to help me, because I couldn't do it alone.

I wanted this battle to be a spiritual journey that would build my children's faith. I wanted them to finish the race knowing that God loves them and is faithful. And can always be trusted to the end no matter what happens in our lives. I wanted them to be equipped for battle no matter what came their way. I wanted them to be filled with compassion for others and someday go out and make a difference in the lives of others who were hurting. I wanted them to have peace and rest in His presence.

The more I understood what I really wanted for my children, I began to accept and realize that the greatest gift I could ever give them would be to totally relinquish them to the Lord. Early one morning, I got on my knees and asked Jesus to forgive me for not honoring Him as Greg and Christie's Creator, Father, and Protector. I acknowledged that they needed their Heavenly Father much more than me. As I ended my prayer, I was ready to begin the relinquishing process in earnest. I knew it was time for me to allow the Lord to grow my faith. A milestone had been reached in my relationship with Him.

Knowing that I had made the decision to trust God and walk in faith, I knew I would have to demonstrate my faith by not only my words, but by my actions as well. I prayed the Lord would guide me step by step in the healing process.

There were days when I thought I was making progress. However, on other days I felt like I had fallen backwards ten steps. I built up a tolerance to some foods and began to put on a little weight. My strength started to return gradually. Because I had cerebral allergies, both my physical and mental health were greatly affected when I came in contact with allergens. As my emotions lead to depression, spiritually I would start doubting what I had always believed about God and His plan for my life.

The part of my immune system that controlled allergies was almost totally nonfunctioning. This left me physically defenseless to fight the intense battle within. It felt I was fighting a war without any weapons to survive.

Though I was surrounded by so many who loved and supported me, I often felt so isolated and alone. Because my illness was difficult to understand, I felt judged and condemned by a few. At times my greatest struggle was the battle within my mind. I was in a fight for my life.

Over the following weeks I ventured out of my room for short periods of time on an occasional basis. I was still imprisoned within the walls of my home, but I was able to sit in our breakfast room for a few minutes every day. Unfortunately, if I stayed too long, the smell of the cedar from the walls prompted an allergic reaction.

My family didn't cook when I was in the kitchen area because the smells made me terribly ill. Even when I was back in my room, they always sealed off the vents whenever they cooked to keep the smells from drifting into my isolation room.

Finally, after many months, I was able to leave my room and sit with my family in the living room for short periods of time—maybe thirty minutes at a stretch—about twice a week. It was wonderful! We would all talk and laugh and try to pretend our lives were somewhat normal . . . until my reactions flared up and forced me to return to my room.

I felt like I was in the process of a rebirth. Having been isolated in my bedroom, I could sense my immune system was rebuilding. Despite frequent setbacks, God was preparing me to re-enter the world. My hope was alive once again. My improvements were no longer driven by my own strong will. Although I was far from being symptom free, I was encouraged by a glimmer of my future being very similar to what I had lived before being diagnosed with Environmental Illness seven months earlier.

Jesus on the Wall

October 22, 1985, began as an ordinary day, but was about to be anything but ordinary!

Around 10:00 that morning, the telephone rang. It was my friend Ann Harris. Always energetic and positive, Ann never let anyone give up, no matter what the problem. Full of enthusiasm, she said, "Linda, the Lord has given me a Scripture for you today. It's Exodus 14:13–14: "Do not be afraid. Stand firm and see the deliverance the Lord will bring you today." She placed extra emphasis on the word today and continued, "The Lord will fight for you, you need only to be still." I thanked her for sharing this passage of God's Word. Little did I know how prophetic that verse would become.

Throughout the morning and early afternoon, I cried out to the Lord. I begged, more earnestly than ever before, for the Lord to give me a sign that His deliverance was indeed at hand. I had no idea what form that sign might take. But I stood in faith that it would come in His way, and in His time.

As the day continued, I kept mentally replaying the words and scripture that Ann had spoken earlier during our telephone conversation.

Father, I am encouraged by Ann's words. I want to believe that you send people into our lives to encourage us and confirm your promises to us. I need to

*know that this message was really from you. God, please fulfill your written word
and give me a sign of reassurance.*

That afternoon I ventured out to the kitchen to sit at the table with
Mom and Grandmother for a few moments. Mom wasn't feeling well. Her
arms were covered with shingles, painful skin lesions caused by a viral infec-
tion. She had a three-inch band of this miserable rash around her waist, as
well. I was convinced that her worry over my condition had aggravated, if
not initiated, her condition.

At about 2:00 that afternoon, Mom said she was feeling tired and left
to lie down. Seconds later, she rushed back to the kitchen. Tears streamed
down her cheeks and she lifted her hands in the air. "Praise God," she exclaimed and wrapped her arm around me. Then she looked me in the eye,
repeatedly saying, "Baby, you're going to be okay. You're going to be okay!"

"Why?" I asked. "Do I get to die?" I knew my words weren't what she
expected. But I was in so much pain and misery, I could not see any way out
other than death.

"Oh, no," Mom responded. "You're going to live. The Lord is going to
heal you."

I stared at Grandmother, who looked as confused as I felt. I stood up
and attempted to calm my mother, holding her hands and taking a step back.

"Please stop crying, Mom," I begged her. "I can't understand a word
you're saying."

We sat down at the table and continued holding hands. Still sobbing,
Mom tried to explain what had just happened to her. "I was lying across
the bed resting, not yet asleep, when I thought I heard a voice speak. 'Hey,'
it said. I looked up, and there on the wall was the Lord's face, just glowing.
He had the sweetest smile and He spoke these words: 'Don't worry, there is
going to be a miracle. Just be patient.' Then He simply disappeared."

I sat there, completely speechless. My heart raced and my spirits soared.

Almost immediately, Satan tried to convince me that it couldn't be
real. My cynical mind came up with an assortment of questions. I grilled

my mother with a long inquisition, but she remained steadfast in her beliefs about the vision.

"Mom," I said, "Jesus doesn't do things like that anymore. You know He didn't really come to you like that. Maybe you were dreaming."

"I wasn't in the room long enough to fall asleep," she replied firmly, which I had to admit was true.

I had always been able to sway Mom a little with my logic and common sense. But no matter how much I tried to convince her that she had not seen or heard directly from the Lord, nothing I said would change her mind. I asked her to repeat the scenario several times to see if her story would change at all. But she never changed a word, not a fraction of an inch.

I continued to interrogate my poor mother throughout the day. I'm sure there were times she wished she'd never told me about the vision!

"Mom, you wouldn't tell me things just to try to make me feel better, would you?"

She shook her head emphatically. "The Lord spoke to me," she insisted, "and no one will ever take that from me." I couldn't convince her any differently. She didn't have to prove anything to me or anyone else. What Jesus had just revealed to her was enough. She didn't have to defend Him or herself. She knew she had heard from Jesus!

I wanted to believe her, but questions and doubts remained. I'd never personally known anyone who actually had a vision. How could it be possible that one would occur in my own home?

The next day Mom came into my room nearly bouncing with excitement. "Look at this!" She thrust her arms in front of me and turned them in all directions. To my surprise, her skin lesions had improved dramatically. "Here, too." She lifted her blouse enough to show me her waist. "The shingles practically disappeared overnight!"

Satan plagued my mind with negative and confusing thoughts. "You know your mother is tired and desperately trying to encourage you. She's so worried about you, now she's creating things in her mind to help you and her cope. You know you're going to stay in isolation forever or die before long."

But as a nurse, knowing how difficult it was for shingles to be cured, I looked at Mom's skin and understood that something supernaturally had occurred. Not only was her skin condition drastically improved, she now had a peace that surpassed all understanding. I was confident that God was in the midst of all that was taking place in my life and the lives of my family members. Excitement began to build within me. I looked forward in anticipation to the days that would follow. My birthday was coming up in a couple of days. As remarkable as Mom's vision had been, I had no idea that the Lord had an even more amazing birthday present waiting for me.

At this point in my journey of faith, I was feeling that God was about to turn my weaknesses into opportunities to demonstrate His love and His power in my life. Little did I know what exactly was in store for me and my family.

CHAPTER NINE

MORE VISIONS, DREAMS, AND MIRACLES

Do not throw away this confident trust in the Lord,
remember the great reward it brings you! Patient endurance
is what you need now, so that you will continue to do God's
will. Then you will receive all that he has promised.
—Hebrews 10:35–36 NLT

TWO DAYS LATER, OCTOBER 24, was my thirty-sixth birthday. No big celebration was planned. I couldn't eat any cake, and the only thing tolerable for me to drink was the special bottled spring water Earl picked up at the Health Food Store.

At 9:30 that morning, as I read the Word of God, I came across John 15:16: "You didn't choose me! I chose you! I appointed you to go and produce lovely fruit" (TLB). As I read, I felt a sense of inner joy and I knew the Lord was speaking directly to me.

Earl came into my room before he left for the office, as he did every day. He knelt beside me as I laid on my aluminum cot, and prayed with me. He gave me a beautiful gold watch for my birthday.

Suddenly, Mom came rushing through the door, crying uncontrollably. I was frightened that something terrible had happened. But she was not upset. On the contrary, she was practically jumping up and down with excitement.

"Now I know you're going to be okay," she said.

"How?" I asked.

"I was sitting in the living room just now," she said, "not really thinking about anything in particular, just looking out the front glass door as I cleaned my glasses. I thought I saw a figure standing at the door, so I quickly put my glasses back on. What I saw was more beautiful and precious than I could ever fully describe. Jesus was standing outside the glass door. I wasn't just seeing things. And it wasn't my imagination. Jesus was standing there in person, glowing. His hands were stretched out as if to say, 'Come unto me, all ye that labor and are heavy laden, and I will give you rest.'"

I immediately recognized the verse from Matthew 11:28 (KJV). I had memorized it years before. A rush of excitement and hope poured through every fiber of my body. I was astonished trying to take in what I just heard . . . too astonished for comprehension. Why would God reveal Himself in such a profound way regarding my healing?

"Then," Mom continued, "in the most loving, gentle voice I have ever heard, He said, 'Don't worry. There is going to be a miracle. Just be patient because I am not through with her yet. I have something special for her to do.' Before I could ask Him anything, He disappeared."

I began to bombard Mom with questions, asking her several times to repeat her story. Each time, I took in every word she had to say and wanted to know more. Had she fallen asleep and had a dream? Did she just think she had seen and heard from Jesus because she so desperately wanted to hear from Him? Had she made up the story in order to encourage me? What did He look like? What was He wearing? When I asked her how she knew that she had really seen Jesus, she looked into my eyes and I knew by the glow on her face that she had, indeed, experienced a visit from the True Healer.

The three of us began to cry as we held each other and prayed. Our hope and spirits soared higher than ever before. We praised God for His faithfulness and confirmation of His plan for my life. My heart was pounding. Excitement overtook me and I praised God for the wonder of it all.

I was determined that this time I was not going to allow Satan to attack my mind and steal my hope. I had to know more about visions and the supernatural.

Confirming the Visions

As soon as Earl left for work and Mom went to take the kids to school, I opened my Bible in the glass reading box and looked up the word "vision" in the concordance. As I looked at the list of references, one verse seemed to leap off the page. It was the first one that caught my eye, even though it was midway through the list: Habakkuk 2:3. I looked it up and found these words: "But these things I plan won't happen right away. Slowly, steadily, surely, the time approaches when the vision will be fulfilled. If it seems slow, do not despair, for these things will surely come to pass. Just be patient! They will not be overdue a single day" (TLB).

I stared at the words "Just be patient." Those were the exact words God had spoken to Mom. I took that as a confirmation from the Lord. I knew He had spoken to us, and that even if my healing was a process rather than instantaneous, it would surely come to pass. I began to gain a new understanding of God. I was convinced that when He had a message for us, He could give us spiritual eyes and ears in order for us to see and hear from Him. My hope was renewed! What greater birthday present could I have ever desired?

My curiosity about visions began to consume my every thought. I pondered Mom's encounters with the Lord and called everyone I could think of to tell them about her visions. I sought everyone's opinion on the matter, although most people appeared uncomfortable with what I told them. Several were speechless, and a few never phoned me again.

I had been raised in great churches, and I had been blessed by these churches in many ways. But the subject of present day visions and miracles was not discussed much. When they were mentioned, I always got the distinct impression that those things only occurred during Bible days. But I was no longer concerned about being identified with any particular denomination or group. I just wanted to know Christ as I had never known Him before. I was determined.

I thought seriously about using the toll-free number for one of the television ministries. I wanted to talk to one of their counselors about visions. For four days I wrestled with placing that call. But every time I started to dial the number, the Lord would say, "Linda, just trust me." He spoke with such authority that I had to be obedient.

After visiting briefly with my family in the living room the following Monday, October 28, at 10:00 in the evening, I decided to go to bed. As I entered the bedroom, the telephone started ringing. A voice on the other end asked to speak to Linda Harriss.

"This is she," I said.

"This is Kathy from the 700 Club."

I couldn't believe what I had just heard. Before she could say anything else, I blurted out, "What are you doing calling me?" I'm sure those words must have sounded very rude, but I was in total shock. After four days of wanting desperately to make contact with this organization, someone from there was asking for me!

She explained. "I kept walking past this table and it had a little piece of paper with your name and number on it. Every time I passed, the Holy Spirit told me to call you."

I then remembered having called in for prayer several months earlier. My exuberance suddenly deflated, I said, "Oh, I see. Your ministry always checks on people who call in."

"We do call sometimes," she explained, "but not always. I called you because the Holy Spirit instructed me to."

This poor woman. I was sure she must have been thinking, *Well, excuse me for calling.*

I apologized for my abruptness and told her all about Mom's revelations from the Lord, and how I had wanted so badly to call but the Holy Spirit had told me just to trust Him instead.

Kathy sounded elated. She assured me with the Scripture from Hebrews 13:8: "Jesus Christ is the same yesterday and today and forever."

"God has given you things like these to hang on to," she said, "because He has a very special plan for your life."

I was bursting at the seams with excitement, hope, and faith!

Two days later I had a conversation with a friend who told me that when "things like this" occurred in her life, she normally kept them private.

My first thought was, *Oh, no, I've blown it. Here I've told the whole world about these miracles, and I was supposed to keep quiet.*

Once again my heavenly Father momentarily calmed me and took away all my confusion and fear. Depression was still raging within, tempting me to relinquish my will to live. The thought of death was still entertaining at times. Early the next morning, the telephone rang and a sweet voice said, "Linda, this is Sandy from the James Robison Association. I'm just calling to check on you."

I'd contacted this ministry to request prayer weeks before. James Robison had a television ministry, but I also knew of him from his days as an evangelist in Houston when he used to hold huge crusades in Texas. Early in my illness, before I got deathly sick, I had attended one of his crusades with Earl, Delores, and Sonny. It was a great service. I really sensed the presence of the Holy Spirit.

My heart moved up into my throat. Should I tell this woman about my miraculous signs and wonders, or should I keep them quietly to myself, as my friend had encouraged me to do?

I decided to take a chance. "Do you believe in visions?" I asked.

Sandy said she did, so I took the next baby step. "Do you think they still take place today?"

She assured me emphatically that visions were definitely for today.

I then told her about all the events that had taken place over the previous few days. "Maybe I shouldn't have told everyone," I ventured. "But I considered my telling everyone simply an act of faith—believing that the Lord God had spoken to me and He will bring His words to pass."

Sandy referred me to that same passage in Habakkuk 2 that God had directed me to earlier, but this time to verse 2: "And the Lord said to me, 'Write my answer on a billboard, large and clear, so that anyone can read it at a glance and rush to tell the others'" (TLB).

I knew now that God had given me a message in a vision, and He wanted me to share it with others! I did wonder, though, why the Lord appeared to my mother instead of to me. As I prayed about this, I realized that He must have known how badly it hurt her to see her child so ill. He wanted to give her peace, and He wanted to use her to be an encourager during this difficult time. And she certainly was a powerful support to me.

The Lord used these things to build my faith, but He also used them to give Mom a confidence she'd never known before. She had truly seen the Master and had heard His voice.

Take Me Out to the Ball Game

I still spent most of my time in my safe room, allowing my immune system to improve by not exposing myself to the numerous things I was allergic to. Dust in the furniture, curtains, and carpet still affected me. And my living room, breakfast room, dining room, and kitchen all had cedar walls. I stayed completely clear of the game room because it was still filled with toxic chemicals from the building materials used to build it several months ago. Some days I felt a tiny bit better and my reactions sometimes were not as severe. This was allowing me to have glimmers of hope. But it sure didn't feel like the miraculous healing had occurred that God had been promising.

My immune system was constantly "up and down" depending on the number of exposures and the amount of time I spent in isolation detoxifying and rebuilding my system. If it rained, there would be a lot of mold in the air. This over-loaded my immune system and my body would react more severely to foods, dust, and the cedar walls. This combination would set me back, and I would have to return to my safe room with the air purifiers.

For weeks I had watched Christie and Greg leave the house for their sports events, and my heart ached seeing the sad look in their eyes. One day at the end of October, I asked Earl to take me to watch Greg play football and Christie cheer. He was hesitant at first, always protective of me.

"The car would have to be completely spotless and dust free," he explained. "Even then, it would be a big risk."

"I know," I said. "But I'm willing to take the chance."

Earl agreed to think about it.

"Whatever you decide," I said, "I'll go along with it." I trusted Earl with such important decisions far more than I trusted myself. I knew I couldn't possibly be objective.

The night before Greg's game, after Earl and I prayed together, we made the decision. I could hardly wait to tell our son the good news. Earl brought him into my room.

"Your dad is going to take me to your game tomorrow," I announced.

Greg's eyes filled with tears. Before he could respond, I warned him about what would be involved. "I'll have to sit in the car under oxygen—no hairdo, no makeup, no nice clothes. Do you think that will embarrass you?"

Greg broke into the biggest smile I've ever seen. He hugged me, and then said, "Mom, I would never be embarrassed. I just want you there."

I watched the clock all the next day. When the time finally arrived, Earl walked me and my oxygen tank directly from my isolation room to my car in the garage. I held my breath as I hurried through the game room. Mom and Grandmother were already in the car. As we pulled out onto the driveway, and then drove down the hill, a sense of excitement flooded my soul. I was outside for the first time since I came home from the hospital! Not really "outside," since I had to stay in the car. But at least I was out of my room.

We headed across town toward the football stadium. As I looked at the cars passing us, I started praying we wouldn't see anyone on the road that I knew. Fat chance of that in a small town like Brownwood. Sure enough, as we approached a stoplight, a car pulled up in the lane next to us. The driver was, of all people, a woman named Starla. She was, without a doubt, one of the most confident, physically fit, and beautiful women in Brownwood. There I was, this insecure, emaciated, haggard-looking person in the car next to her.

I prayed she wouldn't notice me. No such luck. She recognized me right away—I could tell by the shocked look on her face when she saw me through the window. I wanted to dive right into the floorboard. I yanked the oxygen mask off my face and tried to smile. Starla gave me a slight wave. As soon as she pulled away, I put the mask back on. But every time I saw anyone I knew, I repeated the charade.

We arrived at the football field about fifteen minutes before the game. "Let's park on the visitors side," I suggested.

"Why?" Earl asked.

"I don't want anyone I know to see me."

"Babe, we need to be on the home-side."

"Okay," I reluctantly replied.

It didn't take Greg long to spot us. My son was always a great athlete, but he played his heart out during that game. Earl had brought the binoculars, and we all took turns watching Greg and his teammates. I knew most of the boys on the team personally. Many of them had visited our home often.

When Greg's team won the game, I was so proud of them I wanted to jump up and down and holler. I couldn't do that. I just grinned from deep within my heart. Of course, I would have been proud of them even if they lost. For many reasons, it was exciting to watch them celebrate their win. I loved seeing the results of the hard work and discipline the boys had displayed.

After the game, the head coach called the team over to the sidelines, near enough to where we were parked that I could hear his booming voice through the closed car windows.

"There is one player on this team who always gives 100 percent every game," I heard him say. "That person is Greg Harriss." The entire team and coaches applauded. Greg smiled from ear to ear. My eyes filled with tears. I had to believe my son had played that game just for me.

After the game, Earl took me home so I could get back in my clean environment. Then he went out again to pick up Greg. I sat on my cot, absolutely elated. Finally, I was able to almost be a "real mom" to Greg. It was wonderful to feel like a human being again. I literally felt I was experiencing the beginning of a new life.

I didn't feel very well physically. I had tightness in my chest, cerebral swelling, and shortness of breath. But, the discomfort was definitely worth it. And, I wasn't about to tell anyone, because I didn't want them to feel badly for me. I also didn't want anyone to tell me I shouldn't have gone, or that I shouldn't go again in the future!

Christie Cheers

The success of my first trip out made me long for more. I particularly wanted to see Christie cheer. After all, I didn't want her to feel slighted! Besides, I really missed watching her and her friends on the squad.

When Earl and I told Christie that we would be attending her next event, she was excited and hugged me with big tears running down her cheeks. Finally, it was game day. We arrived at the football stadium after the game started so the fans would already be in the stands and not walking by the parking area.

Satan once again was attacking my mind, making me feel ashamed of the person I had become – weak and needy. I hated that I had to hide because I felt so embarrassed by how I looked and the way I had to dress. I didn't want anyone to see the oxygen mask and tank that were in the car for my use. I didn't want everyone to see me as an invalid. I didn't want people to feel sorry for me or pity me. I didn't want others to see that I was totally dependent on my family for meeting almost all my needs. I just wanted my life back. It was grueling being the person I had become. I felt so ostracized by a few people who didn't understand what I was going through. I didn't want to subject myself to further ridicule.

We parked near the end of the lot and couldn't see very well. But I thanked the Lord for the opportunity to be there. Toward the end of the game, Christie and the other cheerleaders walked down to where we were parked. They performed several cheers just for me. I sat there in the car and cried. I had worried that I might embarrass my daughter, being on oxygen and having no makeup, hairdo, or nice clothes. But she couldn't have cared less about any of that. She was just glad her mom was there.

When I returned to my isolation room, I had the same tightness in my chest, cerebral swelling, and shortness of breath like I'd had after Greg's football game. But, again, it was well worth it. At least this night I was encouraged because my reactions were no longer life-threatening and I no longer felt my body was trying to shut down on a daily basis when reactions occurred. Still, I knew that because of the environmental exposures and reactions I experienced, I would have to spend the next few days secluded in my "safe" room in my house. This would hopefully allow my immune system to rebuild. I was encouraged that one day I would return to the life I knew before falling victim to this illness.

Greg's Dream

On November 5 our son Greg went to a weekend church camp with some friends. It was a great experience, and he received many blessings. Three days after he returned, he came to my room first thing in the morning, beaming with a huge smile on his face.

"Mom," Greg said, "I had a dream about you last night. You, Dad, Christie, and I were all sitting in the den when out of nowhere an arrow came flying through the room, barely missing you. A couple of seconds later another one came flying through. But this time it hit you right in the center of the stomach, and you were healed because it was full of the Holy Spirit!"

Greg sat beside me on my cot. "Mom," he said, "I know God was speaking to me and He's going to heal you."

That set my mental wheels in motion, and I started to do some heavy thinking and praying. That evening as I prepared for bed, I passionately prayed, "Lord, I do not want to make something out of nothing. But if Greg's dream was really from you, please let me know by some sort of confirmation."

I awoke early the next morning with the dream still vibrant in my mind. Again I asked the Lord to reveal to me if this was really from Him. That afternoon, Mom went to the post office. When she returned, she handed me my mail. "The printing ink doesn't smell in any of this," she said, "so I think it's probably safe." She offered to get the reading box for me, but I declined, preferring to read without it whenever I could.

Mom left my room and I looked over my mail. Along with several envelopes there was a newspaper from an out-of-town church. I had not subscribed to this church's newspaper, had not received it in the past, and have never received it since. I couldn't imagine who might have sent it to me.

But when I saw the newspaper amongst the envelopes, my eyes almost leaped from their sockets. There, in bold red letters all the way across the top of the page, was one word: ARROW! I was speechless. After taking a deep breath, I shouted for Mom. When I showed her the newspaper, tears filled our eyes. We embraced and gave thanks to the Lord.

When the tears finally subsided, I checked out this "special delivery" more closely. With intense curiosity I read what the pastor had written about how he had chosen the title "ARROW" for the newspaper. The Lord had given him a supernatural vision in the form of a dream. In this dream, God repeatedly gave him 2 Kings 13:17, "The Lord's arrow of victory."

When Mom picked Greg up from school, she told him I had a special surprise for him when they got back to the house. The moment they came home, he rushed into my room.

"Hurry up, Mom," he said, "show me the surprise you have for me."

I smiled. "Close your eyes."

When he complied, I took the newspaper out from under my cot and held it up in front of his face.

"Okay," I said, "Open your eyes."

Greg's face glowed when he saw the newspaper. He grabbed it and stared at it, a joyous grin spreading across his mouth. "See, Mom," he said, "I told you God spoke to me in that dream."

We cried and hugged each other.

"Hey, what's going on in here?" Christie asked when Earl brought her in after returning from school.

Greg showed them the paper and we all celebrated together.

Grandmother's Prayer

Even with God's revelations to me and my family, my healing continued to come slowly. There were still many days when I struggled with severe depression, my brain swelling so badly that I thought it would explode out of my skull, body aches, chest pains, shortness of breath, and other bizarre symptoms. I would feel so useless, as if I was trapped in a body that couldn't exist in the real world. During these days I had to fight to keep from giving up and wanting to die.

God had so often reinforced what I was hearing from Him by making sure I heard it from others as well, but He wasn't done yet. This time, He chose to use Grandmother. She somewhat understood my battle since she was going through her own personal health crisis and had experienced others over her life span. She understood walking in faith and waiting on God's timing.

Grandmother always wanted to be used by God. She wanted desperately to care for me and the family. She had been diagnosed with cancer the year before my illness began and was just finishing chemotherapy when I went into the Houston hospital. As a result of the treatments, her kidneys functioned poorly. They would not allow her to empty her bladder, so it became distended. She spent a great deal of time in severe pain.

On the evening of November 14, when Grandmother was at our home, she began to experience excruciating pain.

"I really need to go to the bathroom," she confessed, "but my old kidneys just won't cooperate."

I encouraged her to go lie down.

"But I feel terrible about not being able to care for you and Earl and the children," she argued.

Finally, her pain (and my persistence) won out, and Grandmother shuffled off to bed. The next morning, she came bursting into my room singing praises to the Lord.

"Grandmother," I asked, "what happened?"

Tears streaming down her cheeks, she explained. "Last night I went to bed, but I couldn't sleep because of the pain. So I cried out to the Lord. I told him how much I wanted to be able to take care of you and the family. I said, 'God, I'm not asking you to heal my kidneys. But, if you can make me well enough to be able to take care of Linda and Earl and the children, I would be forever thankful.' I've never asked the Lord to heal me—just make me well enough so I can care for you."

Earl's mom always had a servant's heart!

"Around 3:00 in the morning," she continued, "I got out of bed because I was hurting so badly and it was time to take my pain medication. But the Lord spoke to me and told me I didn't need the medicine. So I got back into bed. I laid there for another hour or so then decided to get up to see if I could empty my bladder. I started toward Christie and Greg's bathroom. When I got to their dressing room, my lower back—right in the area of my kidneys—started burning like I was on fire. It took my breath away and I couldn't move. The burning sensation was so intense I had to lean over and brace myself on the counter. I sensed the power of God working in my body."

My heart started racing. Grandmother's hands were shaking, but she went on.

"After twenty or thirty seconds of intense burning, I stood up straight and walked into the bathroom."

Grandmother's eyes were clear, the tears gone. "For the first time in months, my kidneys worked like they had never been damaged. They functioned perfectly!"

"Praise the Lord," I exclaimed through my own tears.

"I went back to bed after that and slept better than I have in months."

The next day when Grandmother arrived home from her doctor's appointment she, Earl, and Mom came into my room.

"Hurry and tell me what the doctor said," I exclaimed.

"Hon, all I can say is last night as I cried out to God, He heard my prayer. My kidneys are functioning just fine."

Earl hugged me and held me tight. Our faith had been renewed by the good report. Mom looked at me, struggled to speak as she fought to hold back tears, and said, "Baby, I told you that I heard from the Lord. And I know we can always count on Him to do what He says He is going to do."

The room was filled with so much excitement and emotion. "Lord," I cried, "I feel so overwhelmed by your faithfulness and love. Thank you for healing Grandmother's kidneys and for the blessing she is in our lives."

As Grandmother and I hugged, she looked at me with tears streaming down her cheeks. "He has never failed to answer my prayers and meet my needs. He knew my greatest need was to be able to care for you, Earl, and the children. I'm so happy He made it possible for me to do so."

"Grandmother, God used the healing of your kidneys as a sign to remind all of us that He still performs miracles. On days I'm struggling He gives me assurance that He will be faithful to carry out His promises."

After everyone left the room, I stared out the large bedroom window, looking towards the Heavens, "Lord," I asked, "why would you choose to reveal yourself to me in so many astonishing ways? I will always praise you for what you have done in my life."

We all praised the Lord. Once again He demonstrated His miraculous power in a seemingly hopeless situation. Grandmother's kidneys and hope were renewed. As I lay on my cot just trying to comprehend God's miraculous wonders He continued to perform in our home, I was caught up throughout the day by a sweet voice coming from down the hall.

"Jesus loves me this I know . . . ," she sang. Then she quickly began a moment of praise, "Thank you Lord for healing me. Now I can take care of Linda and the family." A few seconds passed then I heard her whistling "Amazing Grace."

I walked down the hall into the kitchen where she was working.

"Grandmother, I have never heard you sing outside of church or whistle."

"Hon, I am just so happy. Jesus loves me and He extended me His grace."

We both hugged again wiping tears from our eyes.

"Yes, Jesus loves me."

The Harriss family was beginning to gain a whole new understanding of who God is and the miraculous wonders He still performs.

Surrender

From that moment on, my prayers changed. God had demonstrated His love and miraculous power in an unbelievable way. Divine, supernatural intervention! I began to grasp the enormity of His power, mercy, and grace. I began to better understand Him and His Holiness. Seeing Him in His Deity drew my heart towards Him, and I began to feel humbled just realizing how much He loved me.

Suddenly, something deep inside me was drawn to truly knowing him and His presence. No longer did my prayers focus only on healing. Now my heart's desire was, "Lord, I want to know you like I have never known you before." The closer I grew to God, the closer I longed to be.

As I prayed for new direction, God continued to convict me of my need to totally relinquish my life to Him. My mind and my heart were searching for Him as never before. I knew I needed peace. I knew I needed to rest in His presence. I knew that peace would only come at the price of my stubborn self-will.

Throughout the day I prayed, seeking His will for my life. Each time I prayed, I heard Him gently whisper, "I love you Linda. Just trust me." I felt so unworthy of His love because of the many times I wanted to walk away from Him and do everything on my own.

"Lord, I know that I haven't been as grateful, as I should have been for all that you have done for me. I don't even know why you still love me. I am sorry that at times I felt like you didn't love me or really care. I am sorry that I was so consumed with self that I was blinded to the never-ending ways you showed me love."

"Linda," God answered in my heart, "my love for you isn't based on who you are or what you've done. My love for you is based upon who I am. Nothing you could ever do will stop me from loving you. My love for you is unconditional. Simply unconditional!"

The realization of His pure, unconditional love for me was so impactful, I felt compelled to love others unconditionally as He loves me. I knew I was incapable on my own. I needed a heart change. I needed a new heart.

"Father, I offer my heart to you. Reshape it. Remold it. Create within me a pure heart . . . the heart of Christ."

Soon my heart transformation began. I realized and accepted that I would have to love even those who had hurt me. No longer could I base my love for others on feelings. I had to dig deeper into my soul to see others as Christ saw them: imperfect, but lovable, just the way that Jesus chose to see me

I still felt a tug in my heart and soul that there was more He needed from me. As I began digging deeper, searching things that held me back on my quest for total submission, I knew that it was time to release my stubborn will. A strong will had been present in me since birth. I realized that He was asking me to die to self and submit totally to Him. For me . . . that was a seeming impossible test. A test I knew I had to pass.

In my prayers and struggle to die to self, God began awakening me in the middle of the night. I sensed Him saying, "Linda there is still the one thing that I need. You have to totally trust me with Christie and Greg."

Fear consumed me. Panicked, I immediately tried to make a deal with Him.

"You can have every material thing I own. I promise to serve you and even testify of your miracles in my life."

As I continued rambling trying to have it my way, He responded, "Linda, that sound's really good, but I must have your all . . . even your children."

"But, I still can't give you Greg and Christie." I stood firm. I still couldn't release the loves of my life to Him.

As I prayed with this new direction, God continued with even greater conviction to remind me of my need to totally relinquish my life to Him. I cringed at this and wrestled with it in my spirit. I still didn't know how my self-sufficient nature could possibly give up complete control! And yet, more than anything, I knew I needed the peace that only the Lord could give. Finally, I became more and more convinced that this peace would only come at the price of my stubborn self-will.

CHAPTER TEN

TOTAL RELINQUISHMENT

Being confident of this, that he who began a good work in
you will carry it on to completion.
—Philippians 1:6

THANKSGIVING—A NATIONAL HOLIDAY dedicated to giving thanks and eating. I couldn't eat turkey or mashed potatoes or stuffing or yams or cranberries or pumpkin pie. While I didn't want to deprive my family of those delectable delights, I couldn't even stand to be in the same room smelling those aromas. I knew it was going to be a hard day. Sadly, this year my extended family, apart from Dad, would not be coming to our house, because I was allergic to everything and my home was depressing. It was certainly not a fun place to be.

As the holiday approached, my depression became more unbearable.

To make matters worse, the weather changed the week before Thanksgiving and filled the atmosphere with a lot of new pollens that overloaded my immune system. My allergic reactions went crazy, making it harder to tolerate any foods. I again reacted severely to everything else, as well.

"It's been almost a month since you appeared to Mom," I reminded the Lord. "You spoke so strongly to me through your Word. I knew, from all you said, I would have to wait a while to be healed. But surely a month is more than a while."

The enemy played with my mind and emotions, causing me to question again. *"Maybe all the things you think you heard from your God weren't real,"* Satan taunted.

No, I fought in my spirit, *I know I heard from God!*

"Perhaps He's changed His mind," the devil suggested.

God wouldn't do that, I argued.

"Then God is just being cruel to you," my tormentor continued. *"This suffering is too great for any human being to bear."*

Jesus Christ accepted even greater suffering than this when He died on the cross for my sins, I insisted.

"Well, if this is the reward for being a Christian, is it really worth it?" coaxed Satan.

I opened the Word and tried to recall the promises God had specifically given me. I found Philippians 3:10 and decided to try quoting Scripture to the enemy of my soul. I want to know Christ and the power of his resurrection and the fellowship of sharing in his suffering, becoming like him in death.

"Perhaps death is what God wants for you, Linda," Satan persisted.

No, I cried out. *This situation is temporary. It won't last forever.*

"That's true," my enemy taunted. *"Your pain will end . . . one way or the other. You have always been in control of your life. Why not take final control?"*

Final control? I asked. *What do you mean . . . final control?*

"Kill yourself," he said. *"Your husband has guns."*

I was tired of the battle, but most of all I continued to feel so guilty for the pain and losses that I had created for Earl, Christie, and Greg. I felt so badly that their lives had been so disrupted and filled with worry because of me. Maybe if I took my life, then everyone could at some point get back to living life. They wouldn't have to spend their days consumed with me and my illness.

"Of course you will make the ultimate sacrifice, and they will know how much you really love them," tempted Satan.

Ultimate sacrifice? I echoed.

"Yes," my tormentor replied. *"What better gift can you give them than to end their unhappiness. Besides, your agony would end also. And Earl wouldn't have to worry about all of your medical expenses. It would be better for everyone."*

The spiritual battle was so intense. I wrestled with these thoughts day and night.

Suicide

Mom came into my room on the Tuesday before Thanksgiving. I was so depressed I couldn't think straight. The physical pain was unbearable.

"Mom," I whispered, and she drew close to my bedside.

"What do you need, Sweetheart?" she asked, holding my hand. "Whatever you want, I'll get it for you."

"I need . . ." I could barely squeeze the words out of my mouth. "Could you get . . . ?"

Mom leaned closer to hear me better.

"Please give me a gun."

My mother stood up straight and stared at me, obviously upset. "I absolutely will not!" she exclaimed.

"Mom, please," I begged. "I can't keep doing this to my family. I worry that everyone is sad all the time, and we're having to drain our entire savings just to keep me alive. That money was supposed to be for Christie and Greg's college education. I hate what I'm doing to all of you. I feel so guilty."

The enemy had tormented me all day with thoughts about ending my life. *"Earl and the kids will be sad for a while,"* Satan had assured me. *"But no pain could be worse than what you've already created in their lives."* My death seemed to be the best solution for everyone.

"You stop talking nonsense this minute," Mom said firmly. "We have heard from God and He is going to heal you. He has a special plan for your life."

"Everyone is not sad all the time," she said. "Besides, recently we've had a lot of things to be happy about. You've gone on some outings. You're tolerating your foods a little better. I see Greg and Christie with smiles on their faces again. This is just a little setback."

"You're right," I said. "There is a lot to be thankful for." I knew this in my head, but my pain had become so unbearable that my emotions overruled all logic. For several days my head hurt so badly I thought it would explode. Every muscle and joint in my body felt like someone had severely beaten me.

"Waiting on the Lord is so hard," I moaned. "The healing is taking too long. It's not fair to me or anyone else to go on like this."

"Now, that's just your allergic reactions talking and you know it," she said. In truth, some days it was impossible to distinguish between the depression caused by my illness and my real emotions.

Needless to say, Mom told Earl about my odd request. He promptly removed all the guns from the house. My reaction was a deep sense of relief mixed with a lot of confusion. *I'm not alive, but I'm not dead, either. I'm just suspended in midair. I won't kill myself. I don't really want to die. But, I don't want to live the way I am. What am I supposed to do?*

Once again I heard the calming voice of Jesus whisper, *"Just trust me."*

I definitely want to. It's just so hard. I'll try.

On Thanksgiving day Grandmother made the big traditional meal at her house. Earl stayed with me while everyone else feasted. I ate black-eyed peas for dinner. They made me ill.

As soon as Christie finished eating, she came home to relieve her dad so he could go to Grandmother's.

"Greg, Grandmother, and your mom and dad will come up as soon as everyone's done with their meal," Earl promised before he left.

Christie tried to be upbeat, but I could tell it was a struggle for her. My sweet, sensitive daughter had a hard time talking about my illness without crying. So we spoke instead about her basketball games.

"The team's doing really well this year," she said. "We won seven of the ten games we've played so far this season."

I still struggled terribly each time Christie or Greg left the house for one of their sports activities. I hated not being part of their lives. Earl tried so hard to be there for the kids and yet also be with me. I knew he felt stretched in all directions like a roll of salt-water taffy. Mom and Grandmother switched off with him—sometimes attending the kids' events; other times staying with me so Earl could go.

I hated having to have someone "stay with me." I was thirty-six years old, but I had to be cared for like an infant.

Christie sat with me for about an hour before everyone else arrived. After checking in with me, they gathered in the game room to watch the college football games. I looked through my bedroom window and pretended I was at that game. The fantasy provided a temporary escape.

I wondered if I would know how to interact if I ever got out in the world again.

Somehow, I made it through Thanksgiving Day. But I was in for yet another major disappointment.

Gearing Up for Christmas

Traditionally, on the day after Thanksgiving, I always went to Houston to do my Christmas shopping. Sometimes Earl and the kids would go with me. Other times the ladies in the family would enjoy a girls-only excursion.

This year, I sat in my room all day.

We couldn't even have a real tree. My system wouldn't have tolerated the pollen in the house. So on the day after Thanksgiving, Earl and the children went out to pick up an artificial one. Without me, of course. They set it up in the game room, since even the new plastic would have caused a reaction if I breathed the fumes. I watched my family through the long, narrow window near my door. Tears streamed down my cheeks as they unpacked all the boxes of ornaments, garland, and lights.

"Where's the stuff Mom and Mammaw made?" Christie asked.

We had created some decorations out of Styrofoam balls with purple, red, and green sequins, and tiny gold balls held on by gold straight pins. None of these items had an odor, so they were safe for me to handle.

"I don't know," Earl said, a look of bewilderment on his face.

I knew exactly which box the decorations were in. And I could see it on the far end of the room, under the pool table. I tried to tell them, but the Christmas music in the game room drowned out my voice. They couldn't even hear me tapping on the window. I could only watch in disappointment until Greg finally asked, "Is this it?"

Finally, the tree was finished and the boxes cleared away. It looked stunning. And they had done it all without me. I'd always thought that my involvement was vital to the decorating of the family Christmas tree. But there it was. Seven-and-a-half feet of sparkling green evidence that my input wasn't really necessary after all.

The enemy used this scene to remind me once again that my family could survive without me. If I were to leave this world, they would adjust. They would be better off. Yes, suicide was the best gift I could give my family. Knowing that my only weapon against Satan was God's Word, I grabbed my Bible and found 1 John 4:4: "Greater is he that is in you, than he that is in the world" (KJV).

The immediate pressure toward suicide subsided. But I knew, like in the past, the foreboding thoughts would return. I sensed that the enemy didn't want me to live out God's plan for my life. I now began to recognize his schemes. For now, the war within was silent. But I knew it would commence again. Through the power of the Holy Spirit I would be prepared. I would not give in.

Christmas Program

Greg and Christie's school district put on their annual music program in the coliseum. All the choirs from grades seven through twelve participated. Practically the entire community was invited—except me, of course. By this time, everyone knew that leaving my home was not even a consideration.

Christie and Greg came into my room, all dressed up in their Sunday clothes. "You both look wonderful," I said. "I wish I could go with you."

"That's okay, Mom," Christie assured me. "Dad will be there."

I knew she meant her words to be comforting, but they only reminded me of how well my family could survive without me.

Earl and my mom came to get the children to take them to the choir program. "We'll tell you all about it when we get back," Mom promised. "You'll go next year."

Then I heard the front door close and the car drive off down the hill, the house grew deathly quiet. I sat there on my cot, alone and miserable, while my family went off to engage in one of my favorite holiday activities. The whole world was moving on with life as usual, but mine was at a standstill. I was losing touch with all my friends. I was no longer kept in the loop about what was going on. Our worlds were so different and I didn't think we would ever have anything in common again. Depression threatened, but I fought it with all my strength.

Moments later, Rachael, a friend from church, called.

Thank you, Jesus! I really needed a friend in that moment.

"Are you going to the music program tonight?" she asked.

The question ripped my heart open. The answer I had to give broke down my carefully erected fortress of emotional self-protection.

"I wish I could, but I can't," I said, trying to be civil.

"But your children," Rachael said. "They need you. Can't you just push yourself this one time and be there for them?"

Did she think I was just being selfish?

"I know it would be hard, but you've got to get back to living life."

"There's nothing I want more than that," I cried. "But I simply can't do it. My symptoms will go crazy and I'll break down my immune system even more if I leave the house."

"Maybe you need to just trust God and go," Rachael pushed.

"But I can't do those things right now. I did get out to go to Greg's game and to watch Christie cheer. I was able to control my environment. Earl had really cleaned the inside of the car. We have no control over the chemicals that will be used in the coliseum for cleaning. And we can't control the perfumes and scented things people who attend will be wearing."

"I'm under doctor's orders to avoid chemical exposure," I tried to explain as calmly as I could. "He says doing so will keep me from going backwards and might actually speed up my healing process. It takes a lot of discipline, determination, and perseverance to do this. And I'm not just doing it for me. I fight hard to live, every single day, mostly for my family." I stopped there. I didn't want to reveal the thoughts I'd been entertaining of ending the fight for my family's sake.

Once again, I was so hurt by not being understood by people who had no clue how debilitating this illness really is. "If I went to that program, my whole body would try to shut down. I might stop breathing and probably pass out. I'm a lot more concerned about embarrassing Christie and Greg than I am about my reactions."

Rachael was silent for several moments. I prayed my words were sinking in. Finally, she sighed softly, "Well I guess there is nothing I can say that will change your mind. You've always been strong and could do anything. I just thought I could encourage you."

So much for sinking in. If only everyone knew how hard I was fighting.

I knew I had to find encouragement from somewhere or risk falling into a bottomless emotional chasm. I felt like my heart had been shattered by the words that I just heard. I needed a friend. I called my friend Helen. Her children were in college, so I figured she wouldn't be attending the choir program.

The phone rang several times. I rose from my cot and paced the floor a bit. Please, Helen, be home! I needed to hear a friendly voice right now.

As soon as Helen answered the phone, I started crying. I couldn't stop the floodgate of tears.

"What's wrong?" she asked. "Are you all right?"

I didn't know how to explain to her what I was going through. "It's just . . . ," I started. "It's been a long time since you called. I . . . I miss you."

"Well, I miss you, too," she said.

"I wish we could get together again soon, or at least talk on the phone more often." I hated begging for attention from a friend, but I felt desperate. We used to spend a lot of time together when our children played sports together. I missed the friendship. I missed connecting with other parents.

"It's just hard," she replied. "We don't have anything in common anymore."

I leaned against the wall, barely able to maintain my grip on the receiver. I felt like a human pin cushion! Did my friends realize how deeply their words hurt me?

"But for the last few years we played tennis together and had so much fun," I protested.

"Linda, our lives just don't connect anymore. We're just at different places in life."

I was beyond devastated. I felt dead on the inside. I wanted to get mad at her, but I couldn't. She was right. My life was over!

All I could say was, "I guess I'll let you go, then." I quickly hung up the phone. My body slumped to the floor and I cried my heart out.

Sometimes I wished I had a familiar disease. At least people would understand what I was going through. No one understands Environmental Illness. They just think it's all in my head. I hated being so misunderstood. But, how could I expect them to understand? I don't even understand this illness myself.

When I heard my family return home, I pulled myself off the floor, blew my nose, wiped the tears off my cheeks and chin, and stuffed the huge pile of crumpled tissues into the waste basket.

My family doesn't need anything else to worry about. Dealing with my physical problems is enough. They don't need to know about my crazy emotions.

New Year's Eve Wrap Up

A week later, of course, came New Year's Eve. Traditionally, it is time of reflecting over the previous year and making resolutions for improving the next one.

I looked back over 1985. A lifetime had passed since I casually hung up clothes in the laundry room, watched the sunrise, and thanked God for my "perfect" life. After months of confusing allergic reactions, intense pain, deep suffering, and severe loss, my life now had a glimmer of hope. Gone was the constant severe depression that drove me to thoughts of suicide to end my unbearable pain. My struggle to total surrender was in sight. Fortunately, God was patiently abiding with me as I faced my final challenge . . . the relinquishment of Christie and Greg to Him. I still needed just a little time.

That night while the rest of the world celebrated with parties and noise-makers, I lay on my bed, crying out to the Lord. I told Him I still didn't understand what was going on and why all this was happening to me. But I chose to trust Him.

Deep within me I knew this would be a process—one that I prayed would soon be completed.

On New Year's Day I begged Earl to let me have something for dinner besides codfish. I had eaten so much codfish, the very thought of it practically made me nauseous!

A concerned look came into Earl's eyes. "But Babe," he whispered, "fish is the only thing that doesn't make you sick." Suddenly, his expression changed dramatically. "I've got an idea!"

Earl left the room, but soon returned with Greg in tow. Both of them wore heavy parkas and big smiles, and each of them carried an old tackle box.

"What are you boys up to?" I asked.

"We're going fishing," Earl announced with a grin.

"Where? Alaska?"

"No, silly." Greg laughed. "Just to our fishing tank."

"It's really cold out there," Earl admitted, "but we're going to catch some fish for your dinner. Tonight, instead of smelly old codfish, you'll have catfish and bass!"

They each gave me a hug and a kiss on the cheek, then headed out the door. Moments later I heard our old farm truck driving down the hill toward the tank.

I looked out my bedroom window, as I'd done so often in my months of confinement. That big picture window was my link to the outside world, and I spent a lot of time staring out of it—I didn't have much else to occupy my time. I watched the dense fog and drizzling rain and could tell it was bitterly cold out there. A deep sadness enveloped me. I was getting so tired of the fight.

The fishing tank was only a two-minute drive from the house, but my husband and son were gone for almost an hour. Finally, I heard the farm truck chugging up the hill. Earl and Greg came into my room with red noses and cheeks . . . and sad looks on their faces.

"Sorry, Mom," Greg said in a defeated voice. "We really tried, but no luck."

Earl plopped down on his cot and pulled back his hood. "We didn't catch a single fish."

I tried to tell them it didn't matter, that I appreciated their efforts and would gladly go on eating codfish. But that wasn't good enough for my men. We talked about the situation for a few minutes and finally agreed to pray about the fish.

"Let's be really specific in our prayers," I suggested.

We agreed to ask the Lord to allow both Greg and Earl to catch two catfish and two bass.

Earl read Mathew 18:19-20, "Again, truly I tell you that if two of you on earth agree about anything you ask for, it will be done for you by my Father in heaven. For where two or three come together in my name, there am I with them." We each prayed a short prayer, asking the Lord to allow Greg and Earl to catch four fish each. Then they headed back down the hill to the tank.

This time, after only about twenty minutes, I heard the old farm truck coming up the hill. When the garage door went up, I knew the Lord had honored our prayers. The sinks in the garage were where Greg and Earl cleaned their fish!

I sat on the edge of my bed, nearly bouncing in anticipation. Finally, they came into my room, this time with big smiles on their faces. They both talked at the same time, their excitement was obvious.

"Guess what, Mom?" Greg cried.

"You'll never guess," Earl said.

"We caught exactly what we prayed for."

"Exactly!"

"Every time we threw in our lines, we caught a fish."

"Every single time!"

We uttered a quick prayer, thanking the Lord for his faithfulness. Then Greg and Earl hurried out to go clean the miracle fish.

I rejoiced. Once again the Lord had met my needs. He continued to show me that He had everything under control and would take care of me in ways I never dreamed possible. He had every little detail of my life worked out. I was reminded again of the awesome power of prayer.

That night, I ate catfish for dinner. The next night, I ate the bass. My body tolerated both meals exceptionally well and I no longer had to limit myself to codfish! Praise the Lord! I felt like I was seeing more improvement. My mind was clear. The depression was no longer with me every second of the day and I began to imagine myself being able to do the things outside of my home again . . . picking up Greg and Christie, eventually going to their games again, and returning to a somewhat normal life. My hope was building. But I had not received the healing I'd been promised.

I needed a prayer warrior who was committed to praying for the sick. As I prayed for this person, the Lord brought someone to my mind.

Dixie's Prayers

One night in late January, I called a friend of mine named Dixie Dudley. I had known Dixie since the mid-70s when we lived near each other in Pearland. But I hadn't seen or spoken to her in several years, since we no longer lived near each other. I had always considered her a tremendous lady of prayer and faith in the Lord. Dixie would stay up all night praying for people, and often fasted for days if she felt the need was great.

"Dixie," I said, "I've been really sick for a long time with this really strange disease. I sure would appreciate it if you could pray for me, and maybe have your congregation pray for me as well."

For a moment, Dixie said nothing, although I could hear her crying.

"I'm sorry, Dixie," I said. "Is this a bad time?"

"Oh, no," she said. "Quite the opposite. I've been lying here on my couch asking the Lord to give me someone to intercede for."

"Really? Why? Don't you have enough people to pray for already?"

"Several, actually," Dixie said with a sniffle. "But they all died."

Oh, my. Maybe I don't want Dixie to pray for me after all, I thought, mostly kidding.

"I felt called to pray for their healing," she explained, "but more importantly to lead them to Christ. I never offered them anything but the gift of salvation through Jesus Christ."

I sat in silence, not knowing what to say.

"Just three weeks ago," she continued, "one of the people I was praying for, a man named David, died from cirrhosis of the liver after a long bout with alcoholism."

I was beginning to feel embarrassed about having called Dixie. Suddenly, my problems seemed small in comparison to the others for whom she was praying so faithfully.

"After David's death I begged the Lord to allow me the privilege of praying for someone who would be delivered and healed. The minute you told me you were sick, I knew you were the one I'm supposed to pray for."

Now I was really nervous. "Hold on a second, Dixie," I said. I explained to her the details of my illness and how little hope the doctors held out for my future.

She listened attentively as I shared my needs with her. As I wrapped up my story, she started crying again and said, "God has answered my prayers. I'm even more certain now that you are the one He has sent me to intercede for, and I know He is going to deliver you."

A deep sense of faith and hope rose within me. I desperately needed moments like this. In the midst of continually battling my remaining health issue, Dixie's words encouraged me that God had once again used one of His servants to affirm that He would fulfill His promise of healing.

Small But Significant Steps

One night in early February, I laid on my cot longing for the simple things I had enjoyed so much before my illness. I deeply missed being able to pick my children up after school. On rare occasions, they had wanted to ride the bus home with friends. On those days, I would watch the clock and listen for them making their way up our hill. I would greet them in the yard and help them carry their book bags into the house. I would always have a snack ready for them to eat while we discussed their day.

The sound of Grandmother's car pulled me out of my reminiscing. She had picked Christie and Greg up from school and I could hear them driving up the hill. I wanted desperately to greet them all in the breakfast room when they entered the house. I had been particularly weak that day, but I was determined. I pulled myself up off the cot and started down the hall.

"Linda," Mom cried out when she saw me, "let me help you."

She rushed over to me and took my arm. Then she led me, one step at a time, toward the breakfast room.

"I'm okay, Mom," I said, trying to pull my arm out of her grasp.

My mother did not let go. "Baby, you look so wobbly I'm afraid you might fall."

I started to cry. I hated that I had lost my independence. I couldn't even walk by myself!

As we neared the breakfast room, Christie looked up.

"Your mother is real sick and weak today," Mom said.

My daughter looked at us and said, "Mammaw, please let Mom do this by herself. She wants to, and needs to, even if it is hard, or even if it takes a long time to do it." Christie seemed to understand that I was more upset about losing my sense of self-control than I was about my physical weakness.

When Mom looked into my eyes, I gave her a small smile and a slight nod. She hesitantly let go of my arm and I hobbled the rest of the way to the breakfast table. As I lowered myself onto a chair, a small spark of independence surged through me.

Christie and I shared a warm smile, and then Greg launched into a lengthy description of his day at school.

In mid-February, Earl proposed the next step in my recovery. "I think you ought to start getting outside, other than just being in the car."

I reflected on how God had so many times during the last months used Earl as His vessel to speak to me. I reminded myself how God's promises for healing come in dramatic, supernatural ways, but the healing itself was a slow recovery. It wasn't a dramatic supernatural incident at one point in time.

"Where should we go?" I had not been inside a building, other than my own home, since being released from the hospital. For several days, we discussed various options.

One day during the first week of March, Earl came home at lunchtime to give me my allergy shots.

"I've really been praying about when you should start getting out of the house," he said as he administered my injections. "And I decided today is the day!"

I didn't hesitate to agree. I had developed an even deeper level of trust in Earl. Besides, I'd been looking forward to this day for what seemed like forever!

We prayed together about this decision, and both felt God's peace.

Earl secured my oxygen tank on its wheeled cart. I strapped on the ceramic oxygen mask, and Earl checked to make sure everything was working properly. As we headed out the door, I was so excited I felt like a bird finally let out of its cage.

I also felt a bit apprehensive. I wasn't really afraid of getting sick and having a bad reaction. But I didn't want to do anything that might cause my condition to regress, or even to stop progressing. On the contrary, I only wanted to hurry up the healing process!

I stepped out the back door eager to take the walk, but my body was pretty weak. Earl was busy holding my hand and pushing the oxygen cart. I was only able to walk about twenty-five feet before stopping to rest. But I was determined to make it to the small pond at the bottom of our hill, about 100 yards from the house. It took about fifteen minutes due to all the rest stops, but I made it!

"How do you feel, Babe?" Earl asked, his face a mixture of joy and concern.

"I have a headache," I confessed, "but it's not a killer one."

We rested for quite a while alongside the pond. I stared at the path I knew I would have to climb back up. Earl had to almost drag me up the hill, and when I finally got back to the house I was completely exhausted. I immediately went back into my isolation room to detox.

"I can't believe how weak I am," I moaned.

"I'm sure that's partially due to a lack of exercise," Earl said.

"You're probably right." I made a commitment to walk every day, no matter how hard it was. Compared to living in isolation, this seemed a small task. I could take physical pain much better than the emotional kind!

Earl and I started walking to the pond every day at lunchtime. On our fourth walk, when we reached the pond, Earl handed me a rock about the size of an egg.

"What's this for?" I asked.

"To test your strength," he said with a grin. "Let's see how far you can throw it."

I looked across the pond. It was probably twenty-five feet wide. With all the strength I could muster, I tossed the rock toward the opposite side of the water. My arms felt like Jell-O. I hadn't used them for much of anything in almost a year.

The rock dropped into the water no more than five or six feet away.

From that day on, I started exercising my arms by slowly lifting them over my head a few times every day. I also started doing some isometric exercises. I couldn't do many at a time, but each day my arms would stretch a little farther. And each day, the rock would go a little farther across the pond.

"You throw rocks like a girl," Earl teased me one day.

He showed me how to skip rocks like he did when he was a boy. He tossed a flat rock, and I watched it skim across the top of the water, sending out little ripples.

"Let me try," I begged.

My first few attempts failed miserably, and we laughed. It felt wonderful to have something to laugh about again. Soon my competitive spirit won out and I was skipping stones beautifully in no time.

Let Go and Let God

One evening in early February, my friend Susan called and said, "Linda, tonight when I was reading the Word, I found this awesome Scripture that I want to share with you." She read John 16:33 to me: "I have told you these things, so that in me you may have peace. In this world you will have trouble. But take heart! I have overcome the world." God had reminded me of this same scripture earlier in my journey.

"Just think about it," Susan said. "There isn't any problem that God can't handle. Nothing is too big for Him."

That night beside my aluminum cot, I got on my knees on the cold, bare concrete floor and prayed with a passion to hear from the Lord. "Father, this journey has been long and terribly difficult. I am grateful for my progress."

As I knelt there, tears flowed down my cheeks as I brushed them away.

"Lord, is this all just too big – too complicated to fix?"

Silence was all that I experienced. No response. No feelings. No emotions. Only silence. I needed more assurance.

"Please, Lord, Encourage me. I'm trying so hard. But Satan continues to attack my mind and emotions. Empower me to stand against his attempts to take me back to the pit of despair."

I opened my Bible to John 16:33, the Scripture Susan had given me. As I read that verse, I felt a mighty wind rush through me. It took my breath away and I knew it was the Spirit of God. In the touch of a moment, I was reminded that there wasn't a single problem I could ever have that the Lord couldn't handle. It was an incredible experience I knew I would never forget.

For months the Lord continued to speak to me about totally relinquishing my life to Him. But I refused to let go and give Him everything. One night I couldn't sleep because He kept speaking to me, asking me to completely relinquish my life to him. After a couple of hours, I got on my knees and prayed, "Lord, if I am never healed, if I never leave this room of isolation, I want to know you like I have never known you before. Tonight I choose to totally relinquish my life to you."

I continued to earnestly pour out my heart. "Lord, I have finally reached the place in my life where I realize that, more than physical healing, I need spiritual healing and peace."

As I continued to pray, the struggle was still there. I knew deep down what I needed most, but that inner battle was still sparring to override my heart's desire.

"Don't give in," the enemy whispered. *"If you do, you'll be stuck like this forever."*

I countered this taunt out loud. "I have to trust God. He is my only hope."

"A lot of good He has done for you so far," replied Satan.

I fought back, stating, *"Satan, you won't destroy me. God has a plan for my life."*

"It's not a plan that you're going to like," the enemy replied.

Realizing I was in the midst of an ongoing spiritual battle, I began to come against the enemy in the name of Jesus. "Satan, in the name of Jesus you have no authority over my life. You will not destroy me or God's plan for my life."

The room was filled with silence.

I uttered my prayer of relinquishment again. "Lord, if I am never healed, if I never leave this room of isolation, I want to know you like I have never known you before. Tonight I choose to totally surrender my life to you."

I repeated my prayer and waited. A moment later, the Holy Spirit spoke to me again and said, "Linda, you still haven't given me everything. You're still holding on to something."

In my heart I knew exactly what He meant. "No, I responded, you still can't expect me to release Christie and Greg!" A panic rose inside of me with the thought of relinquishing control of my children. I refused to give in. *Not even God could love and protect them like I can,* I thought.

The next two weeks were difficult. I wrestled with the fear of releasing my children to Him. I shared with several of my friends the struggle I was going through and they agreed to pray for me.

The Holy Spirit's dealing with me was intense. I felt His tugging on my heart constantly. Deep inside I knew I needed to trust God completely, but the fear of what He might do with my children was terrifying.

"Lord, what would happen if I totally gave them to you? Would they go through some terrible suffering as I have done. I couldn't bear to see that."

The Holy Spirit continued to deal with me. I tried every way I could to ignore His prompting, but there was no escape.

"Just trust me, Linda, just trust me."

I rationalized and bargained with Him as I pleaded my case. "God, almost everything has already been taken from me, and no mother would give her children away."

"Linda, just trust me," he continued to say.

"But, God, that would be like giving my heart away."

Late one night, I realized that was exactly what I had to do. Since my children were part of my heart, they had to be included in order for me to totally give my all to God. With this revelation, I got down once more on bended knees beside my aluminum cot and prayed.

"Lord, we need to talk," I whispered, not wanting to wake Earl who was asleep on a cot next to me.

"Lord, this is the scariest prayer I have ever prayed, but tonight I am going to trust you with my most prized possessions. Tonight I totally relinquish Christie and Greg to you."

After I prayed, I laid my head on the cot and sobbed tears of relief and joy. With total relinquishment, God was finally able to work in my life. I experienced a new birth, both spiritually and physically. I discovered that I could have the peace I was searching for, whether or not I was healed.

CHAPTER ELEVEN

WALKING IN FAITH

*The Spirit of the Sovereign Lord is on me, because the Lord
has anointed me to proclaim good news to the poor. He has
sent me to bind up the brokenhearted, to proclaim freedom
for the captives and release from darkness for the prisoners,
to proclaim the year of the Lord's favor and the day of ven-
geance of our God, to comfort all who mourn.*
—Isaiah 61:1–2

GOD CONTINUED TO WORK IN MY LIFE. The battle with my health was still
there, as was the battle to walk out the surrender that had been so difficult
for me. But I began to trust Him more as He continued His steady healing
of both my inner turmoil and my Environmental Illness.

Sometimes it seemed like I would progress one step, then fall back
three. I was still taking the shots, but we had reduced the number to about
180 per month instead of the 240 I started with. I was able to tolerate a few
more foods—mainly plain, dry tuna and steamed broccoli and squash—
and I began to put on some weight.

At times I still wondered why God had chosen this journey of faith for
me, and a totally different journey of faith for others who were battling poor
health and wanting to be healed. Pondering these thoughts, I approached
the Lord for answers to the mystery.

Lord, why would you heal me? I know so many children and godly people, who in spite of their prayers for healing, passed on to be with you.

God quickly reminded me, "Linda no one can know the mind of Christ. 'For my thoughts are not your thoughts, neither are your ways my ways.'" (Isaiah 55:8).

I persisted, *But Lord, sometimes I feel guilty when it seems that others who are sick have prayers that appear to be unanswered.*

The Lord answered, *"My child no prayer goes unanswered. You just have to understand that before I created everyone, I knew every day of their lives. The beginning and end. And the journey in between. The greatest healing anyone will ever receive is when they enter into eternity."*

My mind was trying to comprehend all that He had just spoken to me.

"Linda, I'm more concerned with who you or anyone becomes on the journey than what anyone wants out of the journey. Trust me, Linda."

I realized that there were no magic formulas or prayers. It was all about God's plan for my life, and that God had a specific plan for everyone's life. I knew God's love is unconditional and freely and equally given to all. I had to trust Him.

When Earl did our taxes in 1985, he discovered that my medical expenses for the year totaled $27,857.43. The insurance company still refused to pay for any of my treatment because of my diagnosis of Environmental Illness. They continued to claim that no such condition existed.

My doctor, of course, knew better. In mid-February, he insisted I set up an appointment to come in for a check-up. I hated going back to the allergy clinic in Houston. At first, I refused to go. The thought of going back to where I received my death sentence was not somewhere that I ever wanted be a part of again. Just thinking about returning to the clinic caused flashbacks in my mind of devastating medical reports, and people hooked up to IV's looking pale, thin, and awaiting death. I cringed just thinking about hearing patients repeating never ending stories of how they were chemically exposed, and now were diagnosed with Environmental Illness. I wanted no part of any of those things. I just wanted to be healthy again. I wanted my life back.

Even with my loud protest, Earl finally convinced me that it would be a good way to evaluate how much my system had progressed since I left the hospital. I called the clinic and set up the appointment in early March. Dr. Morlen ordered blood work through a lab in Brownwood. This would allow my test results to be returned to him by the time of my check-up.

Earl drove me to the appointment. On our way to the clinic, we passed the hospital where I had been in the isolation unit. An intense sadness overshadowed me and I turned my head and refused to even look.

My visit with Dr. Morlen was routine. He had ordered all the tests that had become so familiar to me while I was in isolation at the clinic. When Dr. Morlen came in with the test results, I searched his face for some sign of surprise at how much better I was doing. I found no trace of excitement or even satisfaction.

"Well, Doctor," I asked, not waiting for him to initiate the conversation, "How am I doing?"

"She's a lot better, wouldn't you say?" Earl added.

"Linda," he said, peering at me over the top of his wire-rimmed glasses, "I did find some improvement in your immune system. I was hoping for even better results. But, I have to remind myself, of how poorly your immune system was functioning, when I first started seeing you."

"But I feel so much better," I said "I know I've made progress."

"You have made progress, but you still have a ways to go.

"So what are you telling us?" Earl's voice trembled.

"Linda still needs to remain in isolation in order to avoid chemical exposures."

"What?" I could not believe what I was hearing.

Dr. Morlen placed his hand on my shoulder. "I'm sorry Linda. I was hoping the results would show more improvement also. But you are not nearly as ill as you were when you first started treatment, nine months ago."

"The Lord has been healing me."

He looked down at the reports. "Sometimes things, including tests, just don't make sense."

I got down from the examination table and fought to hold back my tears, but couldn't. I fell into Earl's arms and he consoled me as he always did.

"Baby, it's going to be alright. We will just continue to believe what we've heard from the Lord."

Dr. Morlen walked up to me and Earl and gently patted both of us on the back. I could see the concern in his eyes, as well.

"Can we please go now," I said. Earl followed me down the hall.

"This doesn't change anything," I told Earl in the car. "I know the Lord is going to continue to heal me."

"I know, too, Babe," he said. But I detected a note of disappointment on his face and a look of sadness in his eyes.

There was no doubt that the treatment Dr. Morlen had provided for me had improved my health. And I was very grateful for his help. But, I knew there was more that I had to do.

Over the next few days, I immersed myself in prayer and the Word. The more I sought the Lord's face, the more assurance I felt that I could believe what He had revealed to me and my family. I had to continue trusting that healing was part of God's plan for my life. Medicine had done its part. Now I had to do mine and walk in faith. God would be faithful to His promises to me.

Venturing Into Once Forbidden Zones

One morning I told Earl that I wanted to try going into the game room.

"Babe," he said, "I don't know if that's such a good idea. You know what Dr. Morlen said."

"I know what the Lord has told me," I assured him. "And I have a real peace about this. Besides, you've been using that ozone machine on the game room every day for months now. With all the ozone that thing has emitted into the air, whatever toxins were in there should surely be neutralized by now."

Earl pulled off the tarps that sealed the game room from the rest of the house.

"Are you sure you're ready for this?" he asked, his hand on the doorknob.

"I'm sure."

Earl opened the door, and then stepped aside for me to enter. When I walked into the room, I just stood there, crying for several minutes.

"Are you okay, Babe?" Earl asked. His face was etched with concern.

I nodded. "I feel like I have fought a battle against every enemy in the world, and the Lord has rescued me, healed me, and delivered me to the other side, to freedom."

We stood in the game room for about fifteen minutes, praying and praising God, trying to comprehend everything that had taken place in our lives. I still had a hard time believing that something so bizarre had happened to me.

I remembered all the people I had met in the clinic and the hospital. I hadn't been able to bring myself to contact any of them, but I knew they could all possibly still be suffering. Even in my moment of triumph, standing in my beautiful game room, I couldn't help but think about those poor women, still in pain, yet still being talked about, laughed at, misunderstood, and judged unfairly. Remembering my own such experiences brought a sharp pain to my heart. But I refused to allow such thoughts to dampen my enthusiasm. I had entered the forbidden room—my own game room—without any adverse reaction whatsoever.

Christie's cheerleading tryouts came up again during spring break from school.

"Mom," she said, "since you're starting to go outside some, do you think you could come to my tryouts?"

I could tell this meant a great deal to her.

"They're going to be held in the high school gym, like always," she added.

I knew the gymnasium would contain innumerable odors. But I couldn't bear to break my daughter's heart again.

"Let's pray about it and ask the Lord to confirm if I should go."

Christie agreed eagerly. I knew she would be praying her heart out. So on the day before Christie's tryouts, Earl and I took our daily walk to the fishing tank and talked about whether or not I should go.

"I think we need to keep praying about it," Earl said, obviously cautious.

Trying not to be impatient or discouraged, I didn't argue and just kept walking.

When we reached the tank, Earl handed me my rock. My heart pounding, I lifted my arm behind my head and threw harder than I had ever thrown before. This time, to my astonishment, the rock made it all the way to the opposite side of the tank. Barely, but it did make it!

Earl and I sat down on the path. We held each other tight, crying and praising the Lord. As we sat there, I uttered a quick prayer and asked the Lord about going to Christie's tryouts the next day. He spoke to my spirit clearly—just as He had done so many times before.

"Go in faith," He said.

I immediately told Earl what the Lord had revealed to me. He agreed it was time I ventured out a little more. When I told Christie, she squealed and jumped up and down. Tears started trickling down her cheeks. She squeezed me so hard; I thought my eyes would pop out!

After giving her a few moments to enjoy the excitement, I asked her the question that had been tormenting my mind all day. "I have to ask you something, Christie, and I want you to be completely honest with your answer."

She nodded, her eyes filled with serious concern.

"I'll . . . have to wear my plain white cotton clothes."

"So?"

"I won't be able to wear any makeup."

"I know."

"And I might have to be hooked up to my oxygen tank."

"Oh, Mom," she said, shaking her head as if I were a silly, worried child and she the parent. "I don't care what you wear or what you look like. And it doesn't matter to me if you have to be hooked up to your oxygen."

"I just don't want . . . to embarrass you in front of your friends."

Christie smiled. "All I care about is that you're there!"

On the day of the tryouts, Christie did a great job. I applauded till my hands were red and sore. I wanted to cheer, but had to bite my lip to keep from bawling.

My presence marked a milestone in our lives. *Thank you, Lord, for allowing me to be here, and for your mercy and grace in my life.*

As soon as Christie finished, Earl and I headed for home. I was only in the gym for about ten minutes, so my reactions were minimal. But at the time, I wouldn't have cared if the experience killed me. My daughter wanted me at her tryouts, and I was thrilled to have been there for her. I cried and praised the Lord all the way home.

In late March, Greg and Christie spent their spring break from school at Mom and Dad's house in my hometown of Pearland, Texas, near Houston. On the second day of their visit, Mom called and told me about a dream she had the night before.

"In this dream," Mom explained, "the Lord healed you. Then you and Earl decided to surprise everyone and drive here without notifying any of us. You made a grand entrance and you were healthy."

I felt so excited, my pulse started to race.

"It gets even better," Mom continued. "When I told Christie about my dream, her jaw just dropped to the floor. I asked her why she was so shocked, and do you know what she said?"

"What, Mom?" In my heart, I knew that whatever I was about to hear would be a confirmation of my mother's dream. Every sign the Lord had given us had been confirmed in some real and miraculous way, and this was going to be no exception.

"Christie told me she had the very same dream on the very same night!"

Mom and I both actually shouted! I'd never been one to yell when I praised God, but this was so amazing. I knew the Lord was confirming to us that my physical healing was His will. I was more confident than ever in God's promise to heal me.

One day in early April, Christie had track practice, but Greg needed to come home right after school. Earl could pick Christie up on his way home from work, but could not leave early that day to get Greg.

"Why don't I go pick him up?" I offered.

Earl panicked. "I don't think it would be a good idea, Babe," he said. "You haven't been away from the house alone."

I took his hand in mine. "I'm really grateful for your concern," I said. "But you can't always be with me to protect me." I saw apprehension in Earl's eyes. "I'll do just fine," I assured him.

Mom and Grandmother were just as concerned as Earl, but I convinced them too. They told me which spot they picked Greg up at each day. As I got into the car, I sensed an exciting feeling of independence. I took no special precautions and didn't even have Earl vacuum the car. I wasn't a bit afraid—God had been faithful to me. I knew the Lord was directing my every step and I could trust Him to lead me.

When Greg saw me sitting in the car, his face lit up with a big, surprised smile. He ran to the car. As he got in, he said, "Mom, I'm so glad you came to pick me up. Can you come get me every day?"

"I sure will try," I assured him. "As often as possible, unless I'm not feeling well."

From that point on, I picked Greg up from school every single day.

My dear friend, Betty, lost her battle with cancer. A few days after the funeral, I got a call from Mrs. Morris, the principal of Early Elementary, where I'd worked before my illness.

"Linda," my ex-supervisor said, "I'm calling to offer you your school nurse job back."

For a moment, I couldn't speak. I was extremely appreciative, but at the same time saddened by the reminder that my illness still had such control over my life. "I'm sorry, Mrs. Morris," I finally said. "I would love nothing more than to be able to take you up on your offer. Unfortunately, the chemicals in the school building would be too toxic for me."

"I am truly sorry that your health is still a problem for you," she said. "And I'm sorry you won't be able to come back to work. We really appreciate the good job you did for the school district the last three years."

As I hung up the phone, I felt a twinge of disappointment. But I was not as upset as I would have been even just a few weeks before. I now knew that God had a plan for my life. I didn't yet understand the details of that plan, but I knew the only place I wanted to be was smack in the middle of His will. That was something I would have said I wanted before the illness but it was far more real to me now after the deep battle I'd been in. I still had doubts and turmoil, but at this time I prayed non-stop that God would help me to stay focused on Him rather than on my illness. I had to rest in His love and compassion.

In my inept attempt to understand what God had done for me, I started to develop a new appreciation for "the little things in life." I even started doing housework again! Mom and Grandmother still cleaned all the floors in my home once a week. One morning as I visited with them at the breakfast table, I announced that I was going to clean the tile floor in the game room that day.

"Now, you don't have to do that," Grandmother protested, getting up from the table as if she intended to tackle the job herself immediately.

"You don't understand," I tried to explain. "I want to."

"Don't be ridiculous," Mom said, standing next to Grandmother. "We don't want you to get sick again."

Somehow I convinced Mom and Grandmother I would be fine and that I didn't need any help. Never had I been so excited about scrubbing floors.

I filled a bucket with soapy water and grabbed a large sponge. I got on my knees in one corner of the room and began the task with a thankful heart. I finally felt like a wife and mother again. I saw each smudge of dirt as a challenge. I was glad to have a challenge in my life that I could actually see, rather than all the unknowns I had dealt with for so long. I knew, if I could conquer this room, I would be ready to take on the rest of the world.

As I cleaned each individual tile, I sang praises to the Lord. I thanked Him for sparing my life and blessing me so much. Over and over, tears pouring down my cheeks, I sang "My Tribute" by Andrae Crouch. I had never felt so grateful to the Lord in all my life. Imagine being ecstatic about scrubbing floors!

When the kids came in from school, I could hardly wait to show off the gleaming game room floor. When they found out I had cleaned it myself, they were thrilled for me.

This incredible victory spurred me on to tackle my next hurdle.

"I want to attend the Sunday night worship service" I announced to Earl. Dr. Don Williford, our pastor, had been extremely supportive, visiting and praying for me and our family during this long journey. I missed his sermons and the fellowship with our church family.

Earl agreed, so a couple of days later, our family made the drive to our church on Sunday evening. As we climbed the stairs to the balcony, I tried unsuccessfully to hold back my tears as I listened to the lyrics of the music playing, "Because He Lives" by Bill and Gloria Gaither. I had sung that song seemingly non-stop during my time of isolation. It brought me peace. It brought me hope. We took our seats and as I lifted my head, with tears still streaming down my cheeks, I made eye contact with Pastor Williford. He had tears flowing down his cheeks and a big smile on his face. We both knew that God had been faithful and answered our prayers.

I'll never forget the joy I felt as we left the service. It was time to get back to life.

A few days later I approached Earl and said, "I'm ready to try to go to Sunday School."

"I'd better call the church, then," he said, "and see if they've sprayed any insecticides recently." We knew they never sprayed in the sanctuary, but our Sunday school class met in the fellowship hall across from the kitchen, where meals were served on Wednesday evenings.

"They haven't sprayed for quite some time," Earl told me after the call. We decided to go the following Sunday. I was so excited!

One nagging thought kept my excitement from being complete. I didn't want anyone to treat me any differently than they used to. But I knew that was too much to ask.

As we approached our classroom, I saw my faithful friends, Kathy, Susan, and Lollie, along with a lot of other people, standing in the hall outside the room.

A woman named Angela, whom I knew only slightly, noticed us first. She interrupted the conversation going on by hollering, "Linda!" Angela rushed over and gave me a big hug. Suddenly remembering why it had been so long since I'd been to church, she pulled away. "Oh, dear," she said in a panic. "I'm probably wearing something you'll react to!"

"Don't worry," I reassured her. "I'm so much better."

"You mean . . . you're cured?"

"Not completely," I had to admit. "There are still some things I react to."

"But she sure is better than she was a few months ago," Earl announced with a big, toothy smile.

Just as we were about to walk into the classroom, Ed walked up to me. Ed was an imposing man, about six-foot-two, with blond hair and a light complexion. He always had an opinion about everything, never hesitated to speak his mind, and had a reputation for speaking before he thought things through.

As Ed approached me, he started laughing loudly. Then, in front of everyone, he said, "Well, Linda what are you eating today? Zebra meat?"

I tried not to let Ed's flippant comment affect me, but I was mortified. As usual, when people said embarrassing things like this, I wanted to run away. I almost started to cry. Several people picked up on my humiliation. Some smiled ruefully as if to say, "I'm sorry." Others winked kindly and shook their heads.

Mary Johnson noticed my discomfort and whisked me away from Ed. "Would you like to share with everyone the amazing things God's been doing in your life?" she asked as we ventured into the classroom. "We could postpone the lesson till next week."

I froze in my tracks. "I couldn't do that."

"Oh, I'm sure Jim won't mind." Mary started toward our Sunday school teacher, but I grabbed her arm to stop her.

"Please," I begged. "I . . . I'm just not ready."

Mary looked at me with eyes full of pity. "Oh," she whispered. "I'm sorry. Of course. I understand."

Once I was safely seated in the back of the room and the attention focused on Jim and the lesson for the week, I was finally able to relax.

Earl kept sneaking sidelong glances at me throughout the lesson. Afterward, he asked how I was feeling.

"It's amazing," I said. "I've had none of my old reactions."

I felt so good, as a matter of fact, Earl and I decided to stay for the morning church services.

Downward and Upward

One evening in early May as we traveled home from one of Greg's baseball games, we got behind a large truck. Its diesel fumes filtered into our Suburban through the air vents. It didn't take long for me to start having chest pains, headache, and depression.

By the next morning, my depression was severe. Earl left for work, and Christie and Greg went to school. Mom and Grandmother took off for the health-food store in Austin, which was 120 miles from Brownwood, to pick up my organic food.

Dad stayed with me, which helped a great deal. He had come up to visit for a few days, and his presence in my room staved off the worst of my depressing feelings. But when he left my room to take a nap, the depression suddenly overwhelmed me. I knew I was going to cry, but didn't want Dad to know how depressed I was. So I grabbed my Bible, tiptoed to the garage, and drove about three minutes to a nearby roadside park on a hill that overlooks our little city. I pulled into a paved area and parked facing our house.

Even before I put the car into park, I started crying. As always, the depression brought feelings of complete hopelessness. I started questioning the Lord and His promises to me, and begged the Lord to let me die.

After sobbing for what seemed like forever, I reminded myself that I couldn't always trust my feelings, but I could always trust the Lord. My emotions were once again out of control due to my allergic reactions, but that did not mean that God had changed His mind or would be unfaithful to me. I opened my Bible and began reading all the Scriptures He had given me during my illness. I felt such power in the Word as I read those verses. My spirits were lifted, and I once again felt hope and a reason to look forward to the future.

When I returned to the house, Dad was waiting anxiously for me.

"I woke up from my nap and you were gone," he said. "I didn't know where you'd gone or what might have happened to you."

I hugged my father, and felt his body trembling. "I'm sorry I worried you, Dad. I just needed to get out for a while."

He wept in my arms, unable to say anything more. I had never seen my father cry before. I was tired and decided to go to my room and rest. Dad walked with me into my room, where he knelt beside my bed. Tears streaking his cheeks, he whispered, "I love you. I'm sorry I was never able to tell you before now."

I had waited my entire life to hear those words. There was never any doubt that my father loved me. But, it wasn't something he ever expressed in words. This illness, even if it resulted in death, would not be too high a price to pay, for the sheer joy of hearing my father say he loved me.

For the next few days I stayed at home, away from the shops and stores in town. I tried to spend as much time as I could stand in my old "safe room." Although the furniture had been moved back in, it still didn't have any carpet or drapes that could collect dust and mold, so the air was the cleanest of any room in the house. My system soon built up again, and I was back on a roll.

A few days later, I told Earl's mom that she no longer needed to come by to help me every day. Grandmother was the type of person who would have cleaned my house until the day she died if I had allowed her to.

"I really appreciate everything you've done for me all these months," I said. "I couldn't have made it without you."

We hugged and cried for a long time.

"Well," Mom announced the next day, "I guess it's time I went back home."

"What?" For some reason, her decision came as a complete surprise to me. It shouldn't have. I'd been doing fine, and she had her own life to live.

Suddenly, I was overwhelmed with the thought of her leaving. I just stared at her, torn by mixed emotions. I was thankful that I could finally take care of myself and my home. But Mom had always been a significant part of my spiritual life, and I hated to see her go. I thought back on all the sacrifices she had made for me, all the big and little things she'd done over the months. Her encouragement, support, belief, and faith in me and in my healing had meant the world to me. It was clear that she was my spiritual anchor. It never mattered if she or someone she loved was going through a personal crisis, her faith always remained unshakable.

Having been raised by this remarkable woman, I was blessed with a considerable amount of faith. But, little did I know when I first became ill, that the strength of my faith would be so severely tested. As I learned the debilitating nature of Environmental Illness I panicked knowing my faith would be hard-pressed in a way it had never been challenged before. I needed someone to stand in the gap for me as I learned that saying you have faith and putting your faith in to action were not necessarily the same. Mom was there when my mind, thoughts, and emotions became cloudy and confused due to the cerebral reactions from foods and environmental toxins.

I couldn't always trust myself to know for sure what I believed or thought, but Mom would pray and believe God would heal me during those times when my raging disease threatened to steal my life away. During those times when I wasn't strong. During those times when I questioned if God really had a plan for my life. I was confident that Mom would see me through this dreadful situation, and she never wavered.

"I'm going to miss having you here all the time," I muttered. As soon as I said the words, I wished I hadn't. I could see in Mom's eyes that she wanted to stay, and that I could convince her to with very little effort. "But you're right, Mom. You should go home and take care of Dad for a while."

"Don't worry," she assured me. "I'll never be more than a phone call away."

"We can even pray together over the phone," I said.

"Absolutely," Mom agreed.

I had surrendered to God, but my deeply ingrained ways of approaching the world hadn't simply disappeared. I was still convinced that I had to be strong. With all the excitement of getting back into the world, teaching Sunday school again, attending all of Christie and Greg's activities, plus managing my house, I once against approached life full-force. Earl and the kids were a great help. But since I carried such a deep sense of guilt about having put everyone through so much, I tried to do everything on my own without asking for help. Besides, the old family adage continued to remind me that I was to be strong and not appear weak. I got busy with activities and constantly exposed myself to things that affected my immune system.

Before long, I began to experience intense symptoms again—tightness in my head and chest, shortness of breath, insomnia, heart palpitations, and depression. I didn't want to give in to these symptoms again, so I chose to ignore the warning signs, although my doctor warned me that I would always have to protect my immune system. Too many chemical exposures would cause a serious relapse. But I refused to believe this would happen to me and didn't want to live in isolation again. I knew the Lord had spoken and I refused to let this illness take me down again.

One morning after Earl left for work and the children went to school, I felt as if my world was crashing in again. My physical symptoms returned and that sense of despair and hopelessness was overcoming me. I went straight to the telephone and called Mom.

When she picked up, I tried to speak but my voice began to quiver and the words just wouldn't come. Finally, I said, "Mom, I haven't been feeling very well the last few days. My system feels like it's trying to shut down again."

"Have you been overdoing things, getting too many exposures to chemicals?"

I admitted that I had. "It just feels so wonderful to be able to do things again that I never want to stop or sit idle." My voice trembled so much I couldn't imagine how my mother was understanding my words, but I pressed on. "Besides, Mom, God said He was going to heal me, didn't He? Do you really believe He will?"

Mom assured me that the Lord would be faithful to His promises. "Remember what He spoke to us on your birthday last year? That the promise He had given would not happen instantly but over a period of time."

Mom and I got our Bibles and read Habakkuk 2:2–3 together: "Then the LORD answered me and said: 'Write the vision and make it plain on tablets, that he may run who reads it. For the vision is yet for an appointed time; but at the end it will speak, and it will not lie. Though it tarries, wait for it; because it will surely come, it will not tarry'" (NKJV). Just hearing the Word brought peace to my spirit once again. I knew that I just had to pull back and take better care of myself.

"Baby, don't be afraid. Just trust Jesus. Listen to Him. Lean on Him to guide you each day. And keep the faith," she said.

"I know, Mom. I'm really trying, but it all just gets so hard."

"I know, but remember we've heard from the Lord. He's going to heal you. He never breaks a promise or goes back on His word," Mom insisted.

"You're right," I said while taking a deep breath.

"Just keep reading the scriptures the Lord spoke to us through," she encouraged.

"I will Mom," I said. "I feel my life is dependent upon them. I just have to continue to trust the Lord."

I knew that God and the allergy clinic had taught me how to take care of myself. I had finally stopped taking the allergy shots. So now I had to pull back and implement what I had been taught. Besides, chemicals were not healthy for anyone. And my body was trying to remind me to avoid them by the reactions that I had.

I was convinced that totally surrendering would be a never-ending process. Day-by-day and step-by-step I would have to humble myself before the Father. He knew my heart. I would trust Him to change my lifelong habits of self-sufficiency to total dependency on Him.

Christ was doing a work in my life. My view of self-sufficiency and my compassion toward others were taking on a whole new perspective. God was preparing my heart. I wanted to understand and support others who were hurting—those who believed no one understood their pain. I wanted to *be there* for them.

One day while lying in bed thinking back over the many experiences I had with the Lord the last year, I found myself with tear-filled eyes.

"Lord," I said, "I feel totally unworthy of the many blessings you have brought into my life."

He replied, *I know Linda, but my love for you is unconditional.*

With tears running down my cheeks, I said, "I don't understand. I have doubted you, been angry with you and thought you didn't love me. I even felt you were punishing me."

The Lord soothed me, *It doesn't matter what you feel or think. You and your circumstances will never change who I am, or my plan for your life.*

"I know. But it's so hard to understand," I cried. "I even wanted to die. And you wouldn't let me. Instead you chose to reassure me, and comfort me."

I had a sense of his gentle presence as I said, "You've listened to my complaints, even complaints against you and yet you've chosen to love and heal me."

As the last words left my lips, I imagined the scene that I had replayed in my mind so many times before . . . that young, little frightened, girl running to Jesus. As He held me in his arms, I felt safe. I felt loved as his tender voice whispered, "Just let me love you. Just let me love you."

As I savored the memory, I drifted off to sleep filled with the peace of Christ that surpasses all understanding.

The first week in August, I got a call from Randy Wallace, the youth minister at our church.

"I was just wondering," he began slowly, "if you and Earl would be up to having the youth group out to your place for a back-to-school fellowship. School activities and pre-season workouts begin in a couple of weeks, and we—"

"I'd love it!" I practically screamed into the receiver.

"You don't have to decide right away. If you want to check with Earl first—"

"I can accept on behalf of Earl and myself," I assured him. Gladly!

He hesitated. "I just don't want to impose. If you don't think you'd be up to it . . ."

"Randy, I want to use the game room for the purpose we had in mind when we built it."

"If you're sure . . ."

"What date did you have in mind?"

"I was thinking maybe the fifteenth?"

"No problem!"

August 15, 1986, was a day of celebration. The game room was packed with kids. Several parents made finger foods and the church provided soft drinks. Randy had a time of devotion and prayer with the kids. Then the game room belonged to the young people. Before long ping pong balls were flying, the juke box was blaring, and the pool table was surrounded by pool sharks.

As I stood quietly in the background observing the group, I praised God in my heart. I was so grateful to be alive and healthy and enjoying what was taking place in this special room that had been dedicated to the Lord to minister to young people.

CONCLUSION

IT'S BEEN MORE THAN THIRTY YEARS since that glorious party in my game room. I'll never forget the elation of seeing that room packed once again with youth who were full of life and vigor.

As I stood in that room full of young people, my mind wandered back to the cool, crisp morning in January of 1985 when that strange, dark voice spoke to me saying, "You're going to have to die. You're going to have to die!" As soon as this thought came to me the Holy Spirit reminded me of Joseph in the Old Testament, who endured years of trials, pain, and struggles. Afterward he said, "You meant evil against me, but God meant it for good in order to bring about this present result" (Genesis 50:20 NASB).

Joseph's words rang true with me. What the enemy had meant for evil, God had used to bring about good. God's healing was a tremendous gift of a second chance at life. But what I later came to understand was that the greatest gifts He gave me were the spiritual riches He blessed me with along the journey.

By far my greatest challenge during those years had been coming to the place of totally relinquishing my life to Christ. It had been easy to give my heart to Jesus as an eleven-year-old. It took my illness, however, to bring me to the point where I finally realized that I was powerless outside of Christ working in me. No matter how much I tried to bring health and healing into my life, my efforts were totally futile. I could do nothing outside of God's power dwelling and manifesting in me through the Holy Spirit. My only hope came through total surrender. No matter the outcome, whether I was healed or remained in isolation forever, I had to trust that the Father would never leave me, and that He loved me. Admitting my weaknesses allowed Christ to bring victory in my life.

Even so, my constant battle for submission and selflessness has been extremely hard. God has continued to strip away layers of pride and self-sufficiency. As I have surrendered my life to Christ again and again, I have seen Him open up the gates of heaven's spiritual blessings of contentment, joy, hope, love, and the assurance of eternity. I have experienced the peace that comes with the surrendered life.

My heart's desire had to become more about honoring Christ for what He had already done for me on the cross than about what I could gain from Him through obedience. My soul had to be filled with gratefulness for the love He demonstrated when He chose to die for me. Gratefulness that He would remain faithful to me. Gratefulness that the joy of eternity with Him would supersede any earthly trials I endured. My constant prayer through the years has been, "Father empower me by your Spirit. Help me to desire holiness more than freedom from the pain of this world."

Another milestone I look back on was the spiritual healing and freedom I received as I forgave those who had hurt me greatly while I battled for my life. In the year or two after my physical health was restored, many times I cried out, "God, how do I get past the harsh comments and lack of understanding I endured during my illness?" His answer was always the same, "By My grace! The same grace I extend to you when you sin against Me!" Through the reflection of the cross, I was able to forgive those who had hurt me so deeply, and in turn, I was even moved to ask forgiveness of those I had hurt myself. I had to accept that the harsh comments came from a lack of understanding my illness. The people who spoke those hurtful words had never intended to hurt me. They loved me. Accepting these truths brought me freedom and comfort.

Spiritual warfare also took on a new meaning for me. The time I spent in isolation and battle gave me a new awareness of how powerful Satan is. I had to make the decision to defeat Satan in the name and power of Jesus. I had to do what Ephesians 6 says and stand on the Word of God.

Put on the full armor of God, so that you will be able to stand firm against the schemes of the devil. For our struggle is not against flesh and blood, but against the rulers, against the powers, against the world forces of this darkness, against the spiritual forces of wickedness in the heavenly places. Therefore, take up the full armor of God, so that you will be able to resist in the evil day, and having done everything, to stand firm. (vv. 11–13 NAS).

God has given us authority to come against the schemes of the enemy—the negative, fearful, discouraging thoughts that Satan plants in our minds and emotions. I had to choose to transform my thoughts, my thinking, and my words. I would no longer allow the enemy to determine truth for me. Truth would be based upon who I was in Christ and His love for me. Accepting this Truth and applying the power that comes God's Word, I was ready to take my life back and live again.

My greatest battlefield with Satan was, without a doubt, in my mind. I had to fight to change my thinking from worldly to spiritual. "Do not conform any longer to the pattern of this world," Romans 12:2 says, "but be transformed by the renewing of your mind," Not only did my thinking have to change, I had to change the words I spoke and refuse to accept words spoken to me that were not whole and healthy. "Death and life are in the power of the tongue" (Proverbs 18:21 KJV).

These powerful, life-changing words became the blueprint for rebuilding my life, and God the Father was the architect of the design. All He was asking me was to have faith in Him and to be faithful to His Word and His plan for my life. These scriptures also became my weapons against the evil one who was determined to destroy me and God's purpose for my life.

Perhaps the most enduring gift from those dark days was prayer, which became my greatest means of hope and inspiration. Prayer ushered me into the presence of the Father enthroned in His kingdom. There my heart and soul connected with His. I was loved. I was understood. I was hopeful. I was never alone. Through prayer He was my constant companion. I stood in the presence of Almighty God. I saw and became confident in the power of prayer. Looking back I can see that every prayer I thought or uttered was answered according to God's ordained plan for my life. Every need met. Every fear overcome. And much needed healing granted for my soul, my mind, my body, and my emotions.

As I finish sharing my journey with you, I don't know where you are in life or what you are experiencing. My prayer is that you will seek God the Father as never before. I pray you will trust Him and allow Him to reveal Himself to you in ways you have never dreamed of or experienced before. I can't promise you healing or that your greatest desires will be fulfilled. But I can promise you that God loves you. No matter what you go through, no matter the earthly outcome, it will all be worth it when you step into the presence of the King of kings, the Lord God Almighty, our Savior . . . JESUS!

I pray that you will trust Christ and live the surrendered life. A life of peace that surpasses all understanding in the midst of the darkest night when all seems hopeless and you are filled with fear. May you always know God's great and perfect love. May you accept Him as your personal Savior. And someday stand in His presence receiving your robe of righteousness and crown of glory. Eternal life!

Paul prayed a beautiful prayer, found in Ephesians 3:14–21, that forms the foundation of my prayer for you:

When I think of the wisdom and scope of God's plan,
I fall to my knees and pray to the Father, the Creator of everything
in heaven and on earth.

I pray that from his glorious, unlimited resources
he will give you mighty inner strength through his Holy Spirit.

And I pray that Christ will be more and more at home in your hearts
as you trust in him. May your roots go down deep
into the soil of God's marvelous love.

And may you have the power to understand, as all God's people
should, how wide, how long, how high, and how deep his love really is.

May you experience the love of Christ, though it is so great you will
never fully understand it. Then you will be filled with the fullness of life
and power that comes from God.

Now glory be to God!

By his mighty power at work within us, he is able to accomplish
infinitely more than we would ever dare to ask or hope.
May he be given glory in the church
and in Christ Jesus forever and ever through endless ages.

Amen.(NLT)

AFTERWORD

PEOPLE WHO DIDN'T KNOW ME when I was going through Environmental Illness are stunned to hear of my journey through a near death experience and Jesus' supernatural intervention. Those who walked with me (or, at times, carried me) through my death-defying journey continue to marvel at God's faithfulness and healing.

Sometimes I wonder if most people react to some form of chemicals, but they are clueless as to the origin of their body aches, pain, mood disorders, insomnia, lethargy, and other physical and mental problems. I pray that in sharing my story people will gain an understanding of the toxic world we live in and the devastating effects it can have on us mentally, emotionally, physically, economically, and even spiritually.

In the aftermath of that 1985 bout with Environmental Illness, I became passionate about making sure others knew of the harmful effects of chemicals in their everyday environments. I began to educate people wherever I could as I told them my story. The changes I urged them to take were the ones I had made in my own life.

I still live in that same house where the illness occurred, but Earl and I have been careful to keep our home environment free from toxins.

If you'd like to begin to decrease the potential effects chemicals can have on you, here are some practical steps I'd suggest you take and a list of toxic products to avoid:

- Eat organic or less chemically contaminated foods.

- Eat certified organic meat. Do not be misled by terms such as: "No added growth hormones," "Natural," "Grass Fed," or "Antibiotic Free." This does not mean the meat is organic or free from chemicals.

- Drink spring water or install a water filtration system in your home to avoid chlorine, pesticides, and other contaminants.

- Avoid plastic containers for storing food or drinks to keep possible toxic chemicals from leaching into your body. Use glass containers.

- Use chemical-free, unscented personal and cleaning products. Deodorants are often very scented and filled with aluminum and other toxic chemicals. Consider trying Tom's of Maine Long Lasting Unscented Deodorant or a similar product.

- Avoid scented fabric softeners and dryer sheets. Replace these by crumpling aluminum foil into a ball (shinny side showing on the outside) and placing it in your dryer as your clothes are drying. Or, you can purchase wool dryer balls or Seventh Generation Natural Fabric Softener Sheets at Target, Walmart, Whole Foods, and various other stores.

- Avoid air fresheners, perfumes, colognes, and other scented products.

- Hair gel and hairspray recipe – Boil 6 ounces of water; add 1 package of Knox unflavored gelatin and stir until dissolved. Allow the mixture to set until cooled down, and then work a small amount into wet hair. You may want to adjust the amount once you are accustomed to using the gel. Dry and style your hair as you normally would. Pour the remaining mixture into an old bottle, maybe an empty hairspray bottle, and spray on your hair as needed. Then pour the gel from the spray bottle into a container and refrigerate, warming the gel when you are ready to use it again. Rinse the spray bottle after each use. This product makes your hair shine and grow.

- Purchase clothing made of natural fabrics. Avoid flame-retardant pajamas for children.

- Purchase organic/non-toxic mattresses and bedding to avoid dangerous chemicals. This is especially important for newborns and young children.

- Do not use standard dry cleaning. Look for chemical-free dry cleaners.

- Use organic pesticides and lawn care products.

- When purchasing a new car, leave the windows down when possible to de-gas the toxic carcinogens (benzene, cyclohexanone, xylene, formaldehyde, toluene, and styrene, among many others).

- Use natural/chemical free products when building or remodeling your home.

Some Everyday Toxic Contributors:
- Cleaning products

- Spray starch – formaldehyde

- Dry cleaning spot remover – solvents

- Oven cleaner – lye aerosols

- Furniture polish – nitrobenzene, naphthalene, phenols

- Silver polish – petroleum products

- Air fresheners – phenol, cresol, ethanol, xylene

- Germ killing disinfectants – creosol, phenol, ethanol, formaldehyde

Personal care products like:
- Toothpaste – phenol, cresol, ethanol

- Cosmetics and mascara – plastic resins, formaldehyde, PVP

- Talcum powder – some contain asbestos

- Aerosol hairspray – PVP, formaldehyde

- Antiperspirants and deodorants – aluminum chlorohydrate, ammonia, formaldehyde

- Permanent press clothing – resins, formaldehyde

- Synthetic fibers – nylon, polyester, acrylic – which are all plastics

Things we use:
- Non-stick pans, ironing board covers, etc. – Teflon: irritant to skin, eyes and respiratory tract

- Insecticides – all kinds

[Reference: Dr. Elson Hass, *Staying Healthy with Nutrition*]

In the years since the 1980s, when Environmental Illness was relatively unknown, research and understanding of the condition has increased dramatically. Now, many people are aware of the chemicals lurking in everyday objects. If you'd like to learn more, see the appendix for a list of resources and practices I recommend.

My health was stable for nearly thirty years, but in 2013 my system crashed again, and I went into another year of battling for my health. The amazing work God did with me there is enough to fill another book. He took me even deeper into my own faith, this time without my mother. That wasn't easy. But I'll never forget what He said to me when the journey began: "Linda, I still have a plan for your life. This time I'm going to grow your faith. In the last journey you relied a lot on your mom's faith. This time it will be your faith that gets you through the battle." And He did take me to a deeper level of faith. This time, the doctors had nothing to offer me. No allergy shots. Nothing. It was just me, Jesus, prayer, the Word, the support of loving friends and family—and God giving me insight into the way He miraculously designed our brains to have the ability to re-wire and restore itself. With a very grateful heart, I continue to be healthy.

What God did in me that second time was more life-changing than the first, and has left me more passionate than ever about sharing His love and the power of prayer. And I want people to become aware of the spiritual battle that we are engaged in each and every day, as well as helping individuals understand the link between our bodies, our minds, and the toxic world that we live in.

RESOURCES

ENVIRONMENTAL TOXINS AND ILLNESS

Books

It's Our Children's Health: Sick Building Syndrome by Janet Hiller, Ph.D.

Is This Your Child? Discovering and Treating Unrecognized Allergies in Children and Adults by Doris Rapp, M.D.

Is This Your Child's World? How Schools and Homes Are Making Our Children Sick by Doris Rapp, M.D.

The Healthy House: How to Buy One, How to Build One, How to Cure a Sick One by John Bower, founder of Ecologically Safe Homes

Whole Green Catalog: 1,000 Best Things for You and the Earth by Michael Robbins and Renée Loux

The EI Syndrome: An Rx for Environmental Illness by Sherry A. Rogers, M.D.

Journals

Well Being Journal
   wellbeingjournal.com

Christian Counseling Today
   AACC.net

Organizations, Physicians, and Websites

Texans for Environmental Health
   txeh.org

Rocky Mountain Environmental Health Association
   bcn.boulder.co.us/health/rmeha/rmehdefn.htm

MCS America – Doctors Treating Multiple Chemical Sensitivity and/or
   Chronic Fatigue/ Fibromyalgia in the U.S.
   mcs-america.org/doctor list.pdf

American Academy of Environmental Medicine
   aaemonline.org

Human Ecology Action League (HEAL)
   ehnca.org

The Environmental Illness Resource
   ei-resource.org

Chemical Injury Information Network (CIIN)
   ciin.org

Fragranced Products Information Network
   fpinva.org/

What You Need to Know about Environmental Medicine,
   by Lisa Nagy, M.D.
   lisanagy.com

Could Multiple Chemical Sensitivity Be the Cause of Your Illness?
   by John R. Lee, M.D.
   johnleemd.com/environmental-illness.html

The Chemical Sensitivity Foundation
chemicalsensitivityfoundation.org

Multiple Chemical Sensitivity: What Is It?
multiplechemicalsensitivity.org

Women's Voices for the Earth
womensvoices.org

PACT Apparel - Organic Clothing
wearpact.com

Safer Chemicals, Healthy Families
saferchemicals.org

Children's Health Environmental Coalition
checnet.org/

Children's Environmental Health Institute
cehi.org/

Environmental Working Group - Safer Cosmetics and Consumer Products
ewg.org

Beautycounter - Safer Skincare
beautycounter.com—beautycounterwithkelsey@gmail.com

e-cloth - Perfect Cleaning with Just Water
ecloth.com

Norwex Products - Cleaning Without Chemicals
norwex.com

Organic/Chemical-free Mattresses
savvyrest.com
toysrus.com (Organic baby crib mattress found on their website)
target.com (Organic baby crib mattress found on their website)

HOW OUR THINKING SHAPES OUR LIVES

Change Your Brain, Change Your Life: The Breakthrough Program for Conquering Anxiety, Depression, Obsessiveness, Lack of Focus, Anger, and Memory by Daniel G. Amen, M.D.

Retraining the Brain: A 45-Day Plan to Conquer Stress and Anxiety by Frank Lawlis, Ph.D.

Switch on Your Brain: The Key to Peak Happiness, Thinking, and Health by Caroline Leaf, Ph.D.

The Healing Power of the Christian Mind: How Biblical Truth Can Keep You Healthy by William Backus

Could It Be This Simple? A Biblical Model for Healing the Mind by Timothy R. Jennings, M.D.

The God-Shaped Brain: How Changing Your View of God Transforms Your Life by Timothy R. Jennings, M.D.

The Brain's Way of Healing by Norman Doidge, M.D.

The Brain That Changes Itself by Norman Doidge, M.D.

The Whole-Brain Child by Daniel J. Siegel, M.D. and Tina Payne Bryson, Ph.D.

How God Changes Your Brain: Breakthrough Findings from a Leading Neuroscientist by Andrew Newberg, M.D. and Mark Robert Waldman

INSPIRATIONAL BOOKS

Flourish by Catherine Hart Weber, Ph.D.

You'll Get Through This: Hope and Help for Your Turbulent Times by Max Lucado

Miracles from Heaven: A Little Girl and Her Amazing Story of Healing by Christy Wilson Beam

Heaven Is for Real: A Little Boy's Astounding Story of His Trip to Heaven and Back by Todd Burpo with Lynn Vincent

90 Minutes in Heaven: A True Story of Death and Life by Don Piper with Cecil Murphey

Fervent: A Woman's Battle Plan for Serious, Specific, and Strategic Prayer by Priscilla Shirer

Hope Heals: A True Story of Overwhelming Loss and Overcoming Love by Katherine and Jay Wolf

The Doorkeeper: Become the Husband and Father God Wants You to Be by Sonny Guess

How to Study the Bible [With the God Who Wrote It] by Connie Willems

ACKNOWLEDGEMENTS

So many people were key to this book:

Connie Willems: I am grateful to have you as my amazing editor and encourager.

Kathy Ide: Thank you for being instrumental in helping me launch this project.

Delores Guess, Hughie Raney, Jr., and Paul Raney: Thanks for always praying and believing in me. I couldn't have made this journey without your love and support. I respect and love you so much. *Blessed to be your baby sister.*

Sally Sue Harriss: Being your mother-in-law is such a blessing. Thank you for your never-ending prayers. I am so grateful that our hearts are united in Christ.

Rick Applewhite: Your love, support, and words of encouragement make me feel honored to be your mother-in-law.

Graham, Raney, Caroline, Wyatt, Lily, Lila, and Luke: Being your Grammy is one of my greatest blessings in life. One of my reasons for writing this book is to serve as a reminder to you that God is faithful: always look for His miracles and answers to your prayers.

Carolyn Pounds and Amy Goodwin: You may have read my manuscript more times than I have. I am so blessed to have you in my life. Thank you for always cheering me on.

Misti Till: Your brilliant mind and sharp eyes played a major role in getting this book ready for print. So thankful for your knowledge and support.

Sandra Raney: Your expertise and help as an English major is greatly appreciated.

Amber Dendy: Thank you for all your love and support throughout this journey. Your belief in me and my story inspired me to never give up writing this book even when I wanted to.

Lisa Wilbanks: I'm appreciative that you always love and reassure me as I attempt new challenges in life. This book was certainly one. Your own personal journey allowed you to connect with mine.

Sonny Guess: Thank you for your visits and praying over me in the midst of your own dark night of the soul.

Peggy Raney: Thank you for always believing that God has a plan for me and this book.

Kathleen Holt: Your friendship, prayers, and encouragement over the years helped keep me motivated to write this book.

Jo Butler: Your inspirational words and prayers of encouragement have helped me to believe in myself and God's plan for my life.

Sharon Holland: I'm so blessed that you kept my office in order in the midst of this project. Grateful for you!

Justin Felts: I don't know what I would have done without you rescuing me from all my computer disasters. You are so appreciated.

Stacy Odom: Thank you for your words of encouragement to write my story.

Anna Ottosen: I'm thankful for your proficient skills used in refining the final details of this book.

Nancy Hill: Thank you for your never-ending words of encouragement to share my story. Your unshakable faith sustained me. I love and miss you!

And my prayer warriors—I am eternally grateful to Judy Lee, Robert Lee, Cindy Evans, Rick Evans, Lindsey Jackson, Mary Jane Ellis, Lynda Waldrop, Faye Jarvis, Kathy Rodgers, Jodie Kennedy, Jennifer Weaver, Adam Holt, Kathy Crowder, Mark Crowder, Margaret Blackburn, Dixie Dudley, Monica Mohney, Judy Guinn, Lisa Marks, Karen Dempsey, Martha Asebedo, LaNell Neill, Carrie Singleton, Kathy Allen, Thresea Williams, Jenny Williams, Denise Felts, Kelly Branham, Ella Burton, Becca

Gifford, my loving family, my church family, and the countless others who have prayed for me, read my manuscript, or encouraged me to write my story.

IN HONOR OF MOM

Peace in the Presence of Angels
August 2011

For the first time, I had to be honest with myself and admit that mom probably was not going to make a complete recovery. I knew I needed to start preparing myself for the day that we would have to part. The thought pierced my heart and shook me to the core of my being. I was torn between seeing her suffer and letting her go.

Mom's number one goal in life wasn't fame and fortune, but loving Jesus and loving others with such Christ-like love . . . so pure, so unconditional, full of mercy and grace. While her journey in life was always about pursuing Jesus, her passion was nurturing and serving others.

As I reflected back over my life, Mom had always been there for me in the good times and in the darkest days. She was my spiritual rock. Years ago when the doctors said I would die, she stayed on bended knees before the Father, on my behalf, begging for mercy and grace. I was determined to do the same for her. I sadly could accept her death, but I struggled with her suffering. I constantly asked the question: Why do godly people have to suffer?

As I looked into Mom's eyes throughout her suffering, I saw peace and acceptance. It was as if she graciously embraced this time in her life as part of God's Eternal Plan. As I saw mom's life coming to an end, I saw her fall more in love with Jesus. She never questioned His purpose in her suffering. Instead she seemed to understand that this necessary season of life would usher her into a Divinely Appointed time without end.

Throughout Mom's suffering, I saw an abundance of God's grace. Grace that was sufficient. Grace that extended into the lives of those of us who loved and supported her during this difficult time. I came to understand that

Mom's suffering was part of the refining process that would prepare her for her eternal home.

During the agonizing time of watching Mom's health deteriorate, I also began to understand that her suffering was allowing me to begin the process of letting go. I didn't want to. I felt guilty. But I knew I had to set aside my own desires to have her with me and accept that God had a far greater plan.

Throughout Mom's battle with cancer, I always told her that I wanted to share in what she was feeling and thinking. I wanted to support her as she had always supported me. I wanted to walk with her through her final journey of faith. I wanted to take away her pain and suffering. But, in spite of my determined efforts, little seemed to change.

Many times I would lie beside Mom holding her as she rested. I pleaded with her to tell me if she was afraid. Her answer was always the same: "I don't have to be afraid. I have Jesus Christ." She spoke those words with such confidence and peace. I needed that same peace. She accepted her fate with such confidence. She was ready to go. I knew I had to give her permission to do so. I needed more time.

I understood that mom had accepted that her days were growing short. She did not see death as the end. She saw it as the beginning of a new life . . . a life of wholeness; a life with the ones she dearly loved. She looked forward to being with Him.

Now it was my time to accept that she would soon pass. I knew it wouldn't be easy, but I was determined to honor Mom's wishes in her final days. I began praying that the Lord would prepare my heart to totally trust her into His presence.

The answer to my prayer came in an unexpected way. One evening, as several of our family members gathered in Mom's room, she began to share with us how, over the last few days, Jesus had revealed to her what was awaiting her in Heaven. We were all eager to hear what she had to say.

Mom gave accounts of seeing her granddaughter, Missy, who had died of cystic fibrosis 29 years ago. She told how Missy was now able to breathe normally and that she didn't have a runny nose. She went on to tell of seeing my dad and how he was so glad to see her. She explained that he told her he had been waiting for her for a long time. She then gave an account of seeing Hughie, my brother, who had died five years earlier. She explained that when she got to the "gate," he was there waiting for her and told her she would love heaven. Her eyes sparkled as she talked about seeing her son. Mom's stories of seeing loved ones in Heaven went on for some time. She told of her heavenly visits with such anticipation. We all looked at each other knowing that Mom had indeed experienced the marvelous accounts that she had shared.

After Mom had given report of her supernatural visits with loved ones, her granddaughter, Lisa, walked across the room and stood at the foot of Mom's bed. Mom kindly whispered, "Lisa, will you please move over. You're standing in front of my big angel and I really like seeing him." Lisa quickly moved. Mom smiled and said, "Thank you. I can see him now." By the way she implied that Lisa was standing in front of her "big" angel, I knew that there were other angels in the room.

Now I totally understood Mom's peace as she walked through the valley of the shadow of death. She was surrounded by a heavenly host of angels.

Never did I question or doubt that Mom had seen our loved ones in Heaven those last few days of her life. Nor did I hesitate to believe that she was in the presence of angels.

I knew as the Father had sent angels to comfort her when she cared for me as I was facing death, He had once again given her spiritual eyes and spiritual ears. I saw that same peace in her that I had seen twenty-six years ago.

As I saw Mom peacefully embrace death, I was finally at peace. I was glad that her suffering would soon be over. As I held her hand and kissed her cheek, she drew her last breath. While my heart was truly broken, I knew her "big" angel carried her into the presence of Jesus as He wrapped her in His arms and said, "Well done, My child."

Mom, thanks for the beautiful memories of a life well lived. Your faith has shaped my life. I am forever grateful. You have now received your Crown of Glory and Robe of Righteousness.

I deeply miss you. But, someday the angels will carry me . . . and I will be with you again.

I love you,
Linda

IN HONOR OF EARL

God's Gift to Me
July 18, 1985

When I think of all the mighty wonders
That my God does command,
My small infinite mind
Can hardly comprehend.
Father, how great is Your love
That You would give Your Son
to die on Calvary
For someone such as Me?
Lord, how I thank you
For all that you have done,
Not just for the big things
But for the little things as well.
Master, there is one very precious gift
That You have bestowed upon me,
And I shall never cease to thank You
For that one so very dear.
He loves me when I'm happy.
He loves me when I'm sad.
This precious gift supports me,
When I'm too weary to stand.
Always at my side to uphold me
When I no longer can stand.
He sustains my faith within me

When my faith seems at its lowest ebb.

God, Your gift tells me I'm beautiful,

When my eyes tell me . . . not so.

Father, oh how he gives me a glimpse of Your love,

By the tender things he says and does.

Your gift holds me so tightly

in his loving arms

During those times when I'm discouraged,

Or when I'm frightened during life's storms.

He holds me when I'm happy,

When all of life is tranquil.

He provides for me a shelter,

Which is more than just a house.

It's a home where Christ abides and lives within our hearts.

This loved one is the father,

Of my precious children from God.

He sets before them an example that is pleasing to your eyes.

And now Almighty Jehovah-Jireh,

I humbly before you stand,

Simply just to praise You,

And thank you for this man.

Happy Birthday, Babe!

I love you and appreciate you with my whole heart!

ABOUT THE AUTHOR

LINDA HARRISS IS REGISTERED NURSE and a licensed professional counselor in private practice in Brownwood, Texas. Linda opened Harriss Center for Counseling in 1994. She counsels individuals and families, many of whom suffer from the effects of mental, emotional, and sexual abuse. Linda is also the author of *Nobody Understands My Pain: Dealing with the Effects of Physical, Emotional, and Sexual Abuse.* She frequently testifies in court as an expert witness on the issue of abuse. Linda's main focus in counseling individuals, is teaching them how to change their lives, through the power and healing that comes by applying God's Word. Part of Linda's role as a counselor is to teach clients how to have a healthier life through healthy eating and living chemically free.

Linda speaks at conferences for churches, schools, organizations, universities, parent, and civic groups. Linda is a member of the American Association of Christian Counselors, Christian Counselors of Texas, American Nurses Association, and The Texas Nurses Association.

Linda and her husband, Earl, have been married since 1969. They have two children, Christie and Greg, married to Rick Applewhite and Sally Sue Wyatt Harriss. They have seven grandchildren, Graham, Raney, Caroline, Wyatt, Lily, Luke, and Lila.

FOR MORE INFORMATION

If you would like further information, please write or e-mail me:

Linda Harriss, RN, MA, M.Ed, LPC
P.O. Box 505
Brownwood, TX 76804
E-mail: Lharriss1@verizon.net

I am available upon request for speaking engagements on the following topics:

- My Personal Testimony

- Living Healthy in a Toxic World

- Experiencing God's Grace

- What To Do with the Hurts You Don't Deserve

- Seeking the Holiness of God

- Establishing a Christ-Centered Marriage

- Experiencing the Power of Prayer

- Abuse—Sexual, Physical, Mental, Emotional

TO ORDER MORE COPIES

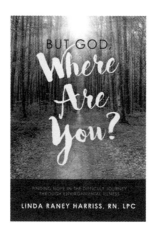

Additional copies of *But God, Where Are You?* may be ordered in the following manner:

- **by mail:** Complete this order form and mail it (along with check, money order or credit card information) to:
  Linda Harriss, P.O. Box 505, Brownwood, TX 76804

- **by phone:** Call (325)646-2155

Name: _____

Address: _____

Phone:# _____

E-mail Address: _____

Please Circle One: Visa   Master-Card

Credit Card #: _____

Expiration Date: _____

CSC # on back of card: _____

Signature: _____

Books can be ordered at the following prices, including tax and shipping:

Number	Cost per book
1-3	$18.95
4-10	$17.95
11+	$15.95

Allow 1-2 weeks for delivery.

Please send _____ copies @ $_____ per book

Total $_____